EAT RACE WIN

THE ENDURANCE ATHLETE'S COOKBOOK

Hannah Grant with
Dr. Stacy Sims Ph.D.

EAT RACE WIN

Copyright © Hannah Grant Cooking and Musette Publishing ApS 2018
www.hannahgrant.com

All photographs are by Hannah Grant unless otherwise mentioned.
Photographs © Hannah Grant
Portrait photos:
Michael Valgren: © Bettiniphoto and Astana Pro Team
Peter Sagan: © Bettiniphoto and Team Bora Hans Grohe
Team Novo Nordisk: © Team Novo Nordisk
Selene Yeager: © Jaime Livingood
Gwen Jorgensen: © Gwen Jorgensen

Art Direction & Design: viction:workshop ltd. | www.victionary.com

viction:ary™

Interviews and Edits: Suze Clemitson
Editor: Musette Publishing ApS
Proofreading and Copy-editing: YuetLin Lim@viction:workshop ltd.

Printed by Colorprint Offset | www.cpo.com.hk
Quality: Taiyang 157g Matt
1st edition, 3rd impression, printed in China 2018
ISBN 978-87-998169-1-0

Other books by Hannah Grant:
The Grand Tour Cookbook
(Danish 2013, Czech 2014, English, German, French 2015)
English: ISBN 978-87-998169-0-3

For upcoming events and more information, please go to:
www.hannahgrant.com
Social media: @dailystews

EATRACE WIN

MUSETTE
PUBLISHING

CONTENTS

Tour de France

July 23rd 1989 – Stage 21

"His heart was pounding and his mind was racing as he continued to press forward. Amidst the noise around him, all he could hear came from within himself: that this was now or never. He had to give it his all to catch the 50 seconds Fignon had on him - the 50 seconds where nothing else mattered.

Having worked so hard to make it back to the top of cycling after being taken out by a gunshot, Greg had to do it. It was the only way, and it was all down to now. His batteries were low, but he had to dig deep to find that last bit of power to finish what would be a historical time trial.

During the warm-up, he had doubted the possibility of making this happen. The tailwind was strong, but Greg had felt incredibly good. His mind was in the right place, so he pushed himself beyond his own limits for the whole 25 km.

As Greg crossed the finish line, his legs were screaming and so was the crowd. He knew he had just done the best time trial of his life, but nothing was settled yet as Fignon had yet to cross the finish line.

Time seemed to pass by in slow motion as the world's eyes were fixed on Fignon, watching the title slip away from him 8 seconds too late. Completely shocked, Greg could not believe it. He had won the Tour at the very last stage, with the closest win ever made. Those 8 seconds were the 8 seconds of victory at the world's most glorious cycling race: the Tour de France."

In 2015, my colleagues from Eurosport and I were at the Giro D'Italia discussing our favorite country for racing, and to this day, my choice remains clear.

Winning the Tour de France had been my goal since I first knew of its existence. It has everything I love: mountains, cobblestones, the summer heat, and the excitement of millions of people lining the roads. The competition is at the highest level of the season, and all of the best riders are there.

Although France is also synonymous with great food, it was unfortunately not so for me when I was a cyclist competing in the Tour. It was very important to provide my body with what it needed to use for fuel, but there were times when I just had to hope that I would be getting enough calories from a tough steak and some overcooked pasta alone.

To that end, I always looked forward to racing in Italy. The food was so good that it made racing easier. There was so much pleasure at the dinner table at the end of a very long day, and it helped me be at my best for the next day.

These days, the top pro teams have professional chefs who travel with them, and I wish that I had been lucky enough to have raced in the Tour de France with a chef like Hannah Grant! Her food is the perfect fuel for anyone, world-class athlete or not; with a focus on actually providing the body with what it needs without forgetting about the pleasure of eating fresh and well-prepared meals in itself.

Healthy living is a crucial factor and foundation when pursuing any goal of any caliber, and I am a firm believer that the right nutrition can make you go further. It is a matter of fueling right and fueling smart, and that does not have to be boring.

Do what you love the most, and do it right.

Greg LeMond

Foreword ····

Dear reader,

First of all, I would like to thank you for picking up this book: a book that is very dear to me and has been in the making for quite some time through some of my life-changing moments. Luckily, these moments have only served to make this book something I am very proud of and excited to share with you.

Over these past few years, I have had the pleasure of working with sports physiologist Dr. Stacy Sims, Ph.D. to create a handbook, guide, and true companion on how to eat throughout the year; for the times when you are training hard, recovering, or even traveling and eating becomes difficult. This book aims to give you all the tools you need to become the best-fueled, energy-packed, lean, happy and winning machine that you can be - and a great cook too.

After all, eating right should not be a punishment!

A word from the author

The EAT RACE WIN Philosophy

The road to personal success in sports as well as everyday living starts with fueling right.

Just as a racecar engine needs the finest fuel to operate at top speed, so does your own engine - your body. Nobody in their right mind would put dirty oil into their Formula 1 car if they were planning for victory, so why should you fill yourself up with junk food or quick-fix, fad-diet meals to fulfill your goals and dreams?

The human body can be trained to achieve incredible performances in running, biking, swimming, and so much more. However, it can never be done without the right focus and dedication combined with eating what is right for you and the physical shape you are in.

Whether your dream is to run 10 km in under an hour, ride in the La Marmotte, complete an Ironman triathlon, or even become a professional athlete one day, you can do anything you set your heart on with the right dietary habits, a healthy body, and effective training.

If you are just beginning to train, do bear in mind that even the best of the best - the top athletes of the world - were also beginners once, and everything started with a dream as well. With this book by your side, you will learn how to fuel right in every season throughout the year, and be at your best to achieve what you have always wanted to achieve.

So, let's get started and make that dream of yours a reality by eating your way to victory.

EAT-RACE-WIN!

Hannah

Intro-duction

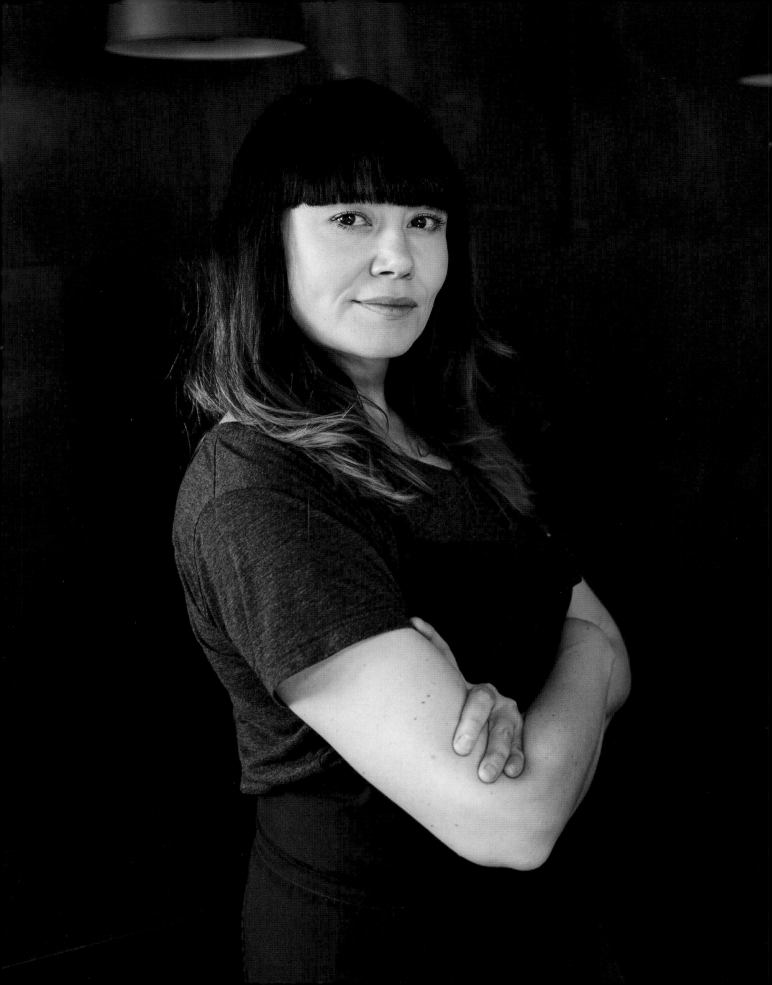

ABOUT HANNAH

Hannah Grant was born in Denmark in 1982 to a Danish mother and Scottish father. Growing up in a loving and creative family filled with people from the theater and restaurant industries, her unique background has served to fire her passion for food, creativity and cooking, which have been her life's work.

After a year spent in the Danish Royal Navy in 2003, Hannah joined a culinary institute in Copenhagen to pursue her dream of combining creative skills and cooking with traveling, all the while continuing to learn, evolve, and develop.

Diploma in hand, she then ventured into some of the best restaurants in the world including the Fat Duck in the U.K. and Noma in Denmark, before the door of opportunity opened to a completely different world of food and endurance sport.

She first spent a year on a kiteboarding expedition boat sailing the South Pacific, where she sourced local ingredients and cooked wholesome meals for the kiteboarders and surfers on board. It was an experience that triggered a new and exciting interest in nutrition, special diets and performance fuel: the start of a unique culinary adventure that shaped her life.

In 2010, Hannah was hired by Bjarne Riis to cook for the riders on his professional cycling team. Throughout the season, she travelled full-time with the team through the incredible culinary touchpoints of France, Italy and Spain.

During her 5 years with them, Hannah also developed a close working relationship with sports physiologist Dr. Stacy Sims Ph.D. The pair clicked instantly and started bringing innovative ideas to the table about fueling endurance athletes at the highest level. It was the start of the process that would end with the publication of the Grand Tour Cookbook in 2013. Originally published in Danish, then translated into English, French and German in 2015, it ended up in the hands of American TV producer, Christof Bove.

Christof took the core themes of the book and translated them into the TV show 'EAT, RACE, WIN' (available on Amazon Prime), which followed Hannah and her crew as they cooked for a cycling team throughout the 2017 Tour de France.

Hannah's culinary experiences in the world of high-performance food have taken her around the globe and yet, her ride has only just begun. She is excited to continue her adventures and share future workshops, master classes, TV shows, and projects with you as they come into being.

Follow Hannah's adventures on **hannahgrant.com**

@hannahgrantcooking

@dailystews

@dailystews

HOW TO USE MY RECIPES

Seasonality and Substitutions

When you are cooking and creating dishes, the best results always come from using ingredients that are in season; when flavors and textures are at their peak, prices are good, and the stock is plentiful.

All the recipes in this book are designed to be flexible with an eye towards the availability of ingredients, where you can easily substitute one type of vegetable for another that is similar. I invite you to play around with flavors and create your own personal versions of my dishes.

Carbohydrates and Starches

Although the recipes in this book mostly focus on proteins, vegetables, and fats, this does not mean that you should not pair them with complex carbs. Instead, you have the flexibility to choose the best types of carbs that work for you, be they baked sweet potatoes, steamed brown rice, or buckwheat noodles. It is entirely up to you to add your preferred starches and tailor the dishes to fit your lifestyle perfectly.

My recipes can also stand alone, in that you can simply prepare them as written without having to add anything supplementary if your activity levels happen to not be at full speed.

Red Meat

When it comes to preparing red meat, everyone has different preferences. With that in mind, you can cook any meat to your liking by making sure that they have reached these core temperatures:

- Rare: 50°C - 53°C
- Red: 54°C
- Medium rare: 56°C - 58°C
- Medium to medium-well: 60°C - 63°C
- Well-done: 63°C+

Resting meat: Always let cooked meat rest for at least 10 minutes before slicing to allow the juices to permeate the meat, rather than ooze out as you slice.

Common Sense

When following my recipes, it is important to always use common sense. For example, you should keep in mind that the density, texture, and water content of different vegetables, fruits, and herbs change throughout the year, and this can affect cooking times. It is always important to keep an eye on food as it cooks, no matter what a recipe says, as some ingredients cook faster than others.

Every oven is different. If you cook frequently and are familiar with the proclivities of your own oven – perhaps yours gets hotter in the upper right-hand corner, for instance – please take this into account. Your oven might be more powerful than mine, or it might cook more evenly. As a result, your dish might be done a little bit before the recipe dictates. Personally, I always make notes in my cookbooks after I follow a recipe, so that I know exactly how to make it perfectly in the future.

Make It Easier: Go Big with Prep and Make-Aheads

While we would all like to have unlimited hours in the day to make time for everything we want to do, life unfortunately does not work that way! Making food and planning meals in advance (including the strategic use of leftovers) will put you one step ahead, give you breathing space in the kitchen, and minimize how long you spend cooking daily.

For example, extra quinoa, potatoes, vegetables, or meat can be used as lunch, a recovery meal, or even a simple dinner the following day. Freeze any extra meatballs for those evenings when you come home late from work and are uninspired to cook. When preparing sauces and dressings, make a larger batch than necessary. You can portion and refrigerate them in sealed bottles. If your fruits are going brown, chop them up and freeze them to make smoothies and desserts anytime. When you start thinking like this, you will be surprised at how much time and money you can save!

More practical tips:

Vegetables such as cabbage, carrots, celery roots, cauliflower, and broccoli can easily be rinsed, cut, and refrigerated raw in an airtight container lined with paper towels on the top and bottom.

Adjust the number of suggested servings per recipe according to your energy output.

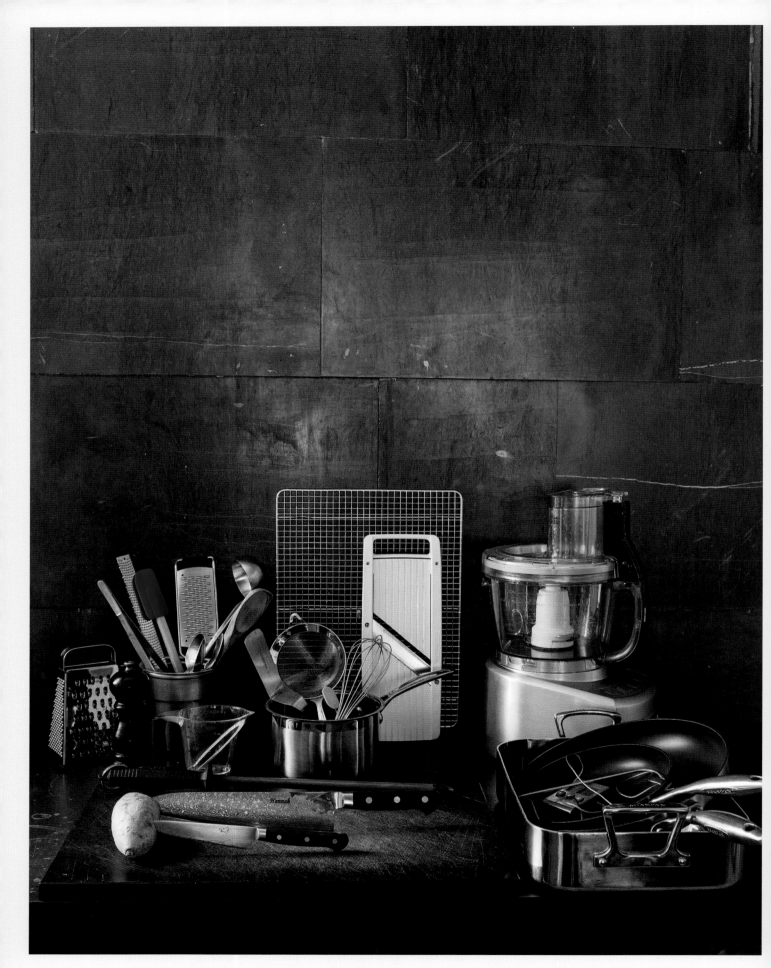

BASIC KITCHEN EQUIPMENT

I am a kitchen tool nerd and have tried almost everything in the market! This is a list of what I think constitutes the perfect basic kitchen set-up. If you have these tools on-hand, it will be easy to prepare all the recipes in this book.

Note: Make sure you invest in good-quality kitchen equipment and tools. If you take good care of them, they will last a lifetime.

- Chef's knife
- Paring knife (also known as a utility or petty knife)
- Ceramic sharpening rod, for sharpening knives
- Peeler – I prefer the diagonal blade ones
- Large cutting board
- Palette knife
- Wooden spoon
- Ladle
- Measure cup
- Saucepan
- Metal whisk with lots of threads
- Heatproof rubber or silicone spatula – medium-sized and flexible
- Graters, both fine and coarse
- Pepper mill filled with black peppercorns
- Meat tongs or pincers
- Japanese mandolin – wide version
- 1 small and 1 large non-stick pan
- Internal meat thermometer with an ovenproof wire or remote control
- Cake tester
- Strainer
- Salad spinner
- Food processor
- Wire rack, for resting meats and cooling baked goods down
- Roasting pan with handles – one that looks good on the table too
- Big chef's pan with a lid – I cook most simmering dishes with this pan

PANTRY ESSENTIALS

A well-stocked pantry holds all the basics for a good meal. This is a list of what you will always find in my pantry.

- Olive oil, for cooking
- Cold-pressed olive oil, for dressings
- Vinegars (apple, balsamic, sherry, red wine, white wine, etc.)
- Salt (flaky sea salt for serving and table/kosher salt for cooking)
- Black peppercorns in a pepper mill (always fresh and not pre-crushed)
- Honey
- Maple syrup
- Toasted sesame oil
- Soy sauce (wheat-free if possible)
- Canned tomatoes
- Dried herbs (oregano, thyme, basil, rosemary, etc.)
- Dried spices (cumin, smoked paprika, coriander, star anise, bay leaves, turmeric, curries, cinnamon, nutmeg, whole cloves, chili flakes, curries of all kinds etc.)
- Parchment paper
- Tin foil
- Plastic wrap (also known as cling film)

Conversion Table

Milliliters (mL) to Cups (C)

Multiply milliliters with 0.004227
E.g. 400 mL * 0.004227 = 1,69 C

Milliliters	Cups
1	0.0042
50	0.21
100	0.42
125	0.53
150	0.63
200	0.85
250	1.06
300	1.27
350	1.48
400	1.69
450	1.90
500	2.11
600	2.54
700	2.96
800	3.38
900	3.80
1000	4.227

Grams (g) to dry Ounces (oz.)

Multiply grams with 0.0353
E.g. 200 g * 0.0353 = 7,06 oz.

Grams	Ounces
1	0.035
50	1.77
75	2.65
100	3.53
125	4.41
150	5.30
175	6.18
200	7.06
250	8.83
300	10.59
400	14.12
500	17.65
600	21.18
700	24.71
800	28.24
900	31.77
1000	35.3

Grams (g) to Pounds (lb.)

Multiply grams with 0.0022
E.g. 800 g * 0.0022 = 1,76 lb.

Grams	Pounds
1	0.0022
50	0.11
75	0.165
100	0.22
125	0.275
150	0.33
175	0.385
200	0.44
250	0.55
300	0.66
400	0.88
500	1.1
600	1.32
700	1.54
800	1.76
900	1.98
1000	2.2

Personalized Recipe Notebook

I keep all of my recipes – with extensive notes beside each of them – in a special recipe notebook. When I am about to prepare a new recipe, I first read through it. Next, I transfer it into my notebook, including all the ingredients and a quick run-down of the steps. The first rule of cooking is that you must know what is about to happen next at all times, so if you read through and transfer a recipe into your notebook, you always will. I learned to do this as a young apprentice cook, after finding out first-hand how important it is to keep all my recipes and notes at hand.

If I have studied and transcribed a recipe, I know exactly how to use it and can tweak or personalize it to my heart's content. I can add ingredients or note how I have changed it, and also document anything that goes wrong (and why). When I cook from transcribed recipes, I am always prepared with everything I need, whenever I need it.

Cooking is a learning process. Like all learning processes, the more you write something down, the better it will stick with you. Perhaps one of the best things about having a notebook is that it will slow the wear-and-tear of your cookbooks. You will have a collection of your favorite dishes with your own personalized touches at your fingertips at all times.

Dietary Symbols

To make it easy for you, these symbols will guide you safely through the recipes.

 Gluten Free

 Dairy Free

 Nut Free

 Vegetarian

 Race Food
Fuel designed for training

 Recovery
Fuel designed for optimal recovery

 Amount of Servings

In Closing

Cooking is an organic process that is never exactly the same twice. Ingredients change – in flavor, water content, density and so on – and you will always have to adjust for this in your seasoning and cooking times. Be present and attentive while you cook. Taste and feel your way through each recipe. The more times you prepare a recipe, the more you will learn about it; and the better you will understand how to tailor it.

Remember: When you fail, you learn best. It takes more than a few tries to be an expert at anything.

Nutrition and Sports Nutrition

BY DR. STACY SIMS

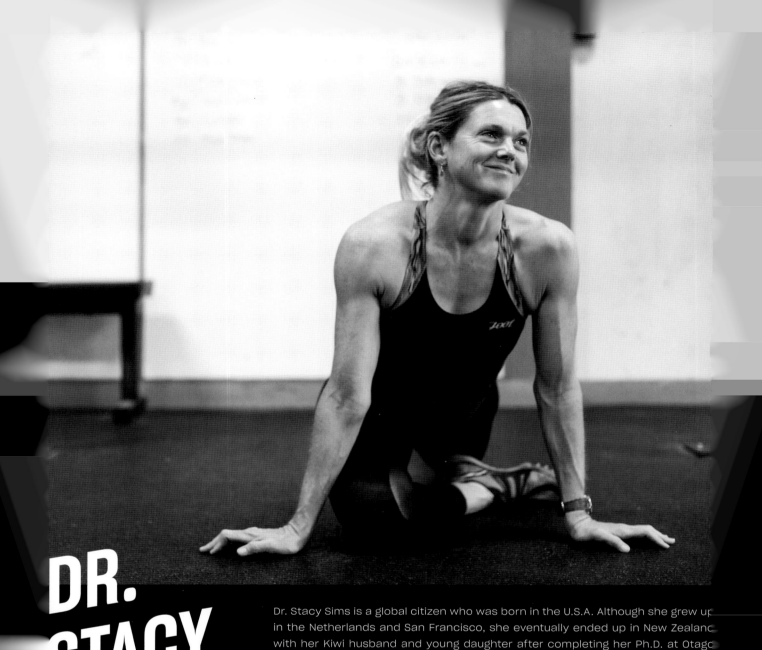

DR. STACY SIMS

Dr. Stacy Sims is a global citizen who was born in the U.S.A. Although she grew up in the Netherlands and San Francisco, she eventually ended up in New Zealand with her Kiwi husband and young daughter after completing her Ph.D. at Otago and her Post Doctorate studies at Stanford; all the while racing her bike at an elite level. Her expertise in nutrition and physiology comes from her research as well as her personal experiences in the peloton, Ironman, and Xterra. She has also worked with a wide range of Olympic and professional-caliber athletes to become who she is today.

As an applied scientist, Dr. Stacy has taken some of her ideas and research to market as consumer products, and has been credited with starting the new revolution in low-carbohydrate functional hydration. In 2012, she was approached by a client/venture capitalist about moving forward with her own company - one that encompassed sex differences, thermoregulation, and hydration in sport. Upon taking the opportunity, she was launched into a whirlwind. Her concept of low-carbohydrate electrolyte drinks and the separation of food from fluid took the sports nutrition industry by storm, challenging the existing dogma and pushing a new niche of products forward. She has since been identified as one of the top 40 women changing the face of the industry, as well as an international expert in sex differences, hydration, and nutrition in sport.

In our modern food culture, there seems to be a disconnect between what it means to be nourished and what it means to be *fed*. In particular, we tend to disconnect training and sports performance nutrition from general nutrition. In doing so, we often rely on engineered sports nutrition products, such as bars, drinks, gels, and powders, to get the fuel we need for training and racing - using 'real food' only for daily nutrition. The effect of this disconnect is widespread: athletes end up eating a diet high in simple carbohydrates and sugars, and end up malnourished with blood markers of metabolic syndrome, *regardless of how much they exercise*.

As humans, we often forget that the body is not linear. It is not an algorithm. It is a complex integration of cellular activity through whole-system interactions. Thus, what we do in our twenties will affect our body composition and long-term health differently than what we do in our thirties. As we age, we find that to keep achieving results, our training and nutrition habits must change.

The goal of this book is to bring nutritious food to the forefront and simplify the process of determining how and what to eat throughout the entire training year. Here, you will learn how to eat low on the food chain while working *with* your body's physiology.

Eat. Race. Win.

Key concepts:

■ There is no such thing as dieting. You must eat real food for nourishment, recovery, training, racing, and health; because health and diet trends usually have nothing to do with maintaining health.

■ Support your local farmers and eat seasonally. The less processed your food is, the more nutrient-dense it is and the fewer 'unknowns' you will consume. Always ask the question: 'Would my grandma eat that?'

■ Health starts with spending time in the kitchen. Invest in your health and spend the time to make simple, nourishing food.

■ Skip the GMOs, pesticides, and additives. Look for recipes and packaged foods with short ingredient lists – lists your grandma would recognize.

■ Listen to your body and nourish it with *real food*. Eat enough of it to get the nutrients you need: supplements are not the answer.

■ Your body changes with the seasons, so the foods you consume during the different seasons should change to meet your biological needs.

DAILY AND SEASONAL BIORHYTHMS: HOW WE CHANGE THROUGHOUT THE YEAR

Biology is an often overlooked but important influence in health and body composition. Your amount of body fat may significantly change over the seasons, particularly in regions distant from the equator where changes in climate, temperature, and duration of daylight are more extreme. As the seasons change, the availability of certain foods will wax and wane; and your eating habits and levels of outdoor activity, physical activity in general, and total energy expenditure will fluctuate.

Some studies have shown that we also have a seasonal fluctuation in weight – one determined that our winter body mass index averages almost 0.5 kg/m2 higher than during the summer. In addition to seasonal differences in weight, potential differences in lipoprotein lipase (LPL) activity and plasma lipids have been shown to vary seasonally. Numerous studies have also demonstrated total cholesterol to be higher in winter than summer by an average of about 4%. Additionally, low–density lipoprotein (LDL) and high–density lipoprotein (HDL) cholesterol levels have been shown to rise in the winter.

Adipose tissue lipoprotein lipase (ATLPL) is a derivative of the lipoprotein lipase enzyme that allows free fatty acids to be stored in fat tissue. Skeletal muscle lipoprotein lipase (SMLPL), a second derivative of the enzyme, pulls fatty acids into muscle to be used as fuel. Studies have found that regardless of fitness level or diet, ATLPL is more active in winter than summer, but only physically active, lean individuals have higher levels of SMLPL activity in the colder months. This finding could mean that a protective mechanism is at work to prevent significant body fat gain in the physically fit.

Food intake and desires also experience seasonal variations. As the daylight hours are reduced and temperatures decrease, the hypothalamus' hunger and satiety centers undergo overt changes. We feel hungrier and crave more nutrient–dense foods, primarily because of increases in the stimulation of fat storage enzymes and production of ghrelin, an appetite–stimulating hormone.

It may seem that these seasonal variations in factors affecting body composition doom us to put on excess body fat, but the body compensates by elevating its resting metabolic rate (RMR) during the cold, dark days of winter. The uptick in RMR has been explained by the effects of melatonin on the hypothalamus. When there is less daylight, more melatonin is produced within the body. This stimulates the hypothalamus' thermoregulation function, thus increasing the body's metabolic rate.

Understanding how the seasonal variations of temperature and daylight hours affect the hormones responsible for metabolic processes allows you to work with your own physiology proactively, including maximizing your food and nutrition choices as you navigate the seasons.

Contemporary Perspectives on Healthy Eating

The new definition of what constitutes healthy food is very different from old-school views. In the past, we've been coached to eat foods low in sugar, fat, and sodium. Today, the focus in on where a food comes from and what is in it. Healthy foods are sustainable – locally sourced, seasonal, and low on the food chain – and minimally processed. How the foods we consume affect our overall health is becoming a theme in preventive medicine. We use healthy food and exercise to promote general health, rather than pharmaceuticals; and the same holds true for sports performance.

The conventional wisdom that exercise can curtail weight and body-fat gain is misleading. You may have heard it a thousand times: "A calorie is a calorie! You need to burn off more than you eat!", but recent research has shown that not all calories are created equal, and that the *types of foods* you eat matter more for long-term health and weight maintenance.

Recent public health research has consistently demonstrated that diets high in simple carbohydrates, white breads, sugar-sweetened beverages, and highly processed foods can be associated with weight gain and metabolic syndrome. Calories from sugar have been proven to affect the body's hormonal control of blood sugar differently from calories from fat and protein. For example, sugar calories promote fat storage and hunger, and fat calories promote a feeling of fullness or satiation. Every additional 150 calories in sugar (about the amount in a can of soda) a person consumes in a day increases the risk of diabetes elevenfold, regardless of how much or how little that person exercises. These results have prompted researchers to re-examine the "eat less, exercise more" dogma. Now, we know that it has more to do with *what* you eat, rather than your total calorie intake.

A 2011 Harvard study was one of the first to closely examine how these factors can be linked to long-term weight gain. Most other research has focused on dieting *after* subjects have gained extra weight. On average, American adults gain at least a pound per year, so the effects of the extra weight on a person's general health a few decades on can be significant.

These researchers tapped into findings from three large, on-going studies – the Nurses' Health Study, the Nurses' Health Study II, and the Health Professionals Follow-Up Study – that have followed more than 120,000 adults who were free of obesity and chronic diseases at the beginning of the studies.

These studies uniformly found that the standard American diet (SAD) was not helpful in keeping off the pounds. For example, over a four-year period, a daily serving of French fries was associated with 3.35 pounds of weight gain, and daily consumption of potato chips was associated with an additional 1.69 pounds. In fact, white potatoes were found to be among the biggest dietary offenders, followed by sweetened soda (a 1-pound gain every four years) and processed and unprocessed red meats (about a 0.95-pound gain across the same time period).

All Calories Are Not Created Equal

Conversely, the studies found that increased consumption of several specific foods, namely, vegetables, fruits, nuts, and whole grains, was associated with notably lower instances of weight gain. Effectively, this dispels the myth that all calories are equal. Nuts are calorie-dense, but their consumption was in fact associated with weight loss. Whole and reduced-fat milk were also associated with weight loss, despite their significant differences in caloric content. Thus, it is surprising that a 150-calorie bag of potato chips, something with considerably less calories than nuts, milk, and many other whole-food items on the Harvard researchers' list, could be linked to significant weight gain.

No laws of thermodynamics are being broken here. As the Harvard researchers wrote: "Differences in weight gain seen for specific foods and beverages could relate to varying portion sizes, patterns of eating, effects on satiety, or displacement of other foods or beverages." That is, potatoes and white bread may be less satisfying than unprocessed, higher-fiber foods with the same number of calories. Eatings foods that have lower levels of satiety increases hunger signals in the brain and encourages more food consumption, thus the total number of calories consumed will rise.

Foods high in fiber, on the other hand, take longer for the body to digest, and thus make you feel full for a longer period of time. Eating more of these foods displaces more processed foods from your diet. Thus, if you eat more fruits, nuts, vegetables, and whole grains, you will gain less weight over time.

Where does all this leave old-school teachings about carbohydrates, fats, and proteins, and how does this relate to my training and performance? Between fears about high-protein diets, high-fat diets, and diets heavy in really *any type* of carbohydrate, athletes have become utterly confused about what and how to eat.

Essentially, the most significant factor in figuring out the proper metrics for your health and performance is not your training or your Training Stress Score (TSS); instead, it is your diet. Certainly, your training and exercise are very critical to your performance, health, and body composition, but if your fuel is terrible, your body still will not function the way you want it to. To clear up some of the stress, let's take a closer look at what the functions of carbohydrates, fats, and proteins in your diet really are.

Carbohydrates: Are They the Devil on Your Shoulder?

There has been an uptick in interest in "anti-Western" diets recently, with a movement towards the increased intake of higher-fat, higher-protein, and lower-carbohydrate foods. In these diets, the *kinds* of food you eat matter as much or more than the macronutrient aspects. This is most evident in paleo and gluten-free diets and in the eat-local, sustainable-farming movement.

In addition, interest is high these days in using nutrition and nutrient-intake timing as a method to improve health, wellness, and sports performance. Debate rages on about the efficacy of low-carb and low-grain diets, for example, and their relationship to athletic performance.

"But wait," you might think, "I have heard that low-carb-high-fat diets are awesome for performance." The answer is yes, sort of. Low-carb diets increase fatty-acid oxidation during exercise and promote intramuscular fat storage (hey, your body is smart; if there is not enough primary fuel to support the stress it is under, it will go for a secondary sourc; in this case, fat, and store more of it for use the next time it encounters the same stress). However, this does not necessarily translate into improved performance, as it ends up compromising your ability to maintain high-intensity and/or prolonged exercise. No matter what side you take in the great carbohydrate debate, facts are facts: the body needs carbohydrates in order to exist, and it specifically needs highly accessible carbohydrates to perform well in the world of cycling and endurance sports.

I would like to take you back to some basic physiology before diving into the ins and outs of lower-carb diets and endurance performance. First, let's talk about the role carbohydrates play in providing energy for working muscles, providing fuel for the central nervous system (CNS), enabling and perpetuating fat metabolism, and preventing the use of protein as a primary energy source. Remember, carbohydrates – specifically glucose – are the preferred source of energy for muscle contraction and biologic labor.

Glycogen, which is the term for glucose in its stored form, is limited in its ability to be stored: about 350 g in the muscles and 40 g to 50 g in the liver of a non-obese 70 kg man. The glycogen stored in a particular muscle is used directly by that muscle during exercise; glycogen cannot be "borrowed" from resting muscles. Hence, it is critical to restore glycogen levels in the muscles of the endurance athlete.

The minimum daily intake of carbohydrates necessary for survival – that is, for supporting the CNS, red blood cell production, the immune system, and all tissues dependent on glucose – is ~130 g. You need considerably more than that to support any physical activity or exercise.

The intensity and duration of an exercise period will directly affect the amount of glycogen that is used. It is common knowledge that low-intensity exercise (e.g. 20% to 30% maximal oxygen update [VO2 max]) uses minimal glycogen, but when the intensity of an exercise period approaches ~75% of VO2 max, the body's storage of muscle glycogen will be almost completely depleted within 2 hours of cycling. It is interesting to note that the rate of glycogenolysis is higher in Type IIa and IIb muscle fibers at intensities greater than 75% VO2 max (usually, Type I fibers are depleted first). Thus, in a race situation, when it is "go time" from the very start, the actual rate of total muscle glycogen depletion will be faster, thus increasing the probability of early fatigue. It appears that glycogen availability is the primary limiting factor on sustaining intensity during prolonged exercise, and that the initial amount of glycogen stored in the muscle is directly proportionate to an athlete's ability to sustain work rates greater than 70% VO2 max over time. Since dietary carbohydrates are a significant contributor to muscle glycogen stores, and thus to performance, there is most definitely a time and a place for carbohydrates in an athlete's diet.

Why is that? To put it succinctly: your diet *can* and *should* include some processed carbs as fuel during training, but the bulk of your carbohydrates should come from eating fruits, vegetables, and whole grains as part of your normal diet.

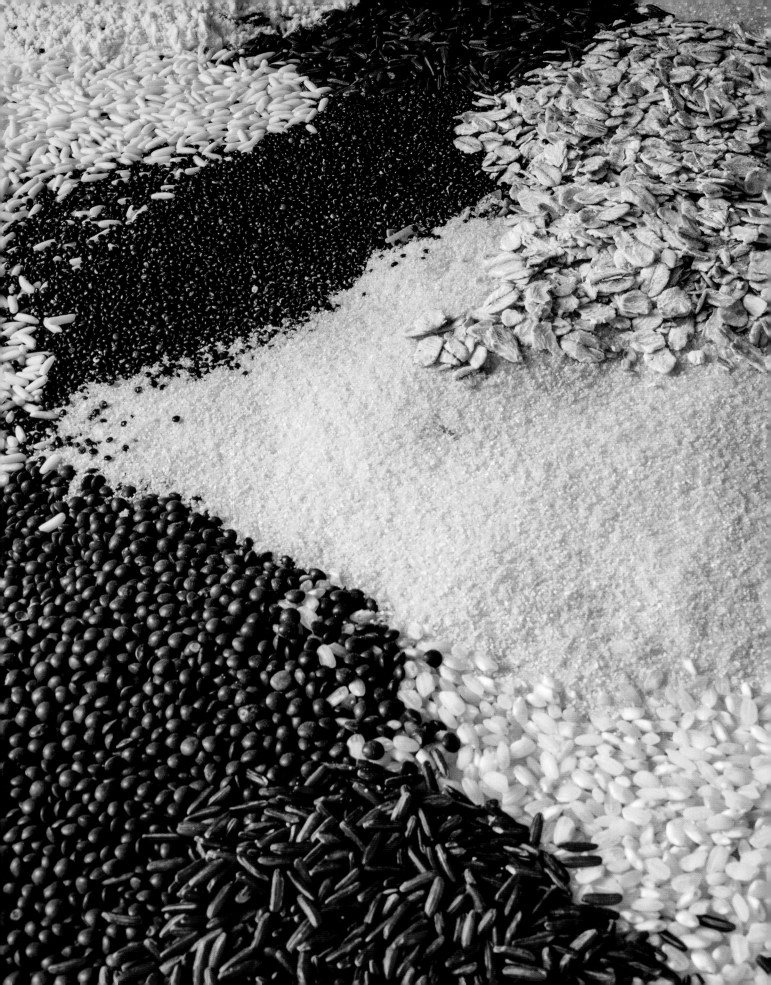

CARBS 101: SIMPLE VS. COMPLEX

Carbohydrates are made up of sugar molecules, which your body breaks down into fuel, especially when you are working hard. Sugars, starches, and fiber are all basic forms of carbohydrates. There are two main types of carbohydrates: simple and complex.

Simple Carbohydrates

Simple carbohydrates include table sugar, syrup, and glucose. Most of the time, these carbs should be avoided (exception: in training foods) and are conventionally recognized as "bad" carbs. You can also include candy, cake, beer, and cookies on this list.

Complex Carbohydrates

Complex carbohydrates include foods such as oatmeal, apples, berries, carrots, quinoa, and other whole grains. For a long time, people believed that complex carbohydrates were universally better for you than simple carbohydrates, but that is not always the case.

You see, your body treats complex and simple carbohydrates alike. It breaks them down into usable sugar energy to fuel your muscles and organs. It is not the type of carbohydrate that really matters; instead, it is how quickly your body can break it down and how much it will spike your blood glucose levels.

That said, it is not as simple as dividing complex carbs from simple ones. The Glycemic Index (GI) is a slightly more sophisticated way to rate the quality of carbohydrates. The GI classifies foods according to how quickly they break down in the body and how high they boost blood sugar levels. However, bear in mind that neither low-carb nor low-GI diets are a magic pill for fat loss. Your focus instead should be on eating the right amount of healthy foods to fuel your metabolism, which in turn will help you burn fat.

The important thing to remember is that your body needs carbs, even if fad diets tell you otherwise. *This becomes even more important if you are engaged in intense exercise.* Without carbohydrates, your body will begin to break down your muscle tissue to fuel your body, which will sabotage your efforts.

It is just as important to note that the health benefits of low-carb diets do not mean that they are strategically better for fat loss. Research published in *The American Journal of Clinical Nutrition* dropped a bomb when it compared a lower-carb diet to a higher-carb diet and discovered that each yielded no significant difference in rates of fat loss, metabolism, or lean mass retention.

DITCH THE LOW-FAT IDEA

Fats do not make you fat! For a long time, fats were thought of much like carbs are today, and blamed for every health problem imaginable. It is the reason why for nearly 20 years, "low fat" was synonymous with healthy.

Many still follow this theory to determine if something is good for them: "If it is low fat, it has to be good." Others believe that if a food does not contain saturated fat, it is okay. Much like any other silver-bullet nutrition solution, this simply is not true. As overall fat consumption decreased among Americans, its levels of obesity increased, according to Centers for Disease Control and Prevention (CDC) data. This was due to a variety of factors, including frequency of meals and snacks, size of meals, and consumption of sugar.

So, what is the bottom line on fat? Fat is good. For starters, fat is an essential nutrient for many biological processes, and it is something most endurance athletes simply do not eat enough of. It plays an important role in helping the general functioning of your body. It is a critical coating for nerves that speeds up and facilitates conduction of messages, ensuring that every neurochemical signal that is sent from your brain through your body is communicated efficiently.

Types of Fats

■ **Monounsaturated fats:** Monounsaturated fats are found mostly in high-fat fruits, such as avocados, as well as nuts, like pistachios, almonds, walnuts, and cashews. This type of fat can also be found in olive oil. Monounsaturated fats help lower levels of bad cholesterol and raise levels of good cholesterol. They have also been shown to help fight weight gain and may even help reduce levels of body fat.

■ **Polyunsaturated fats:** Like monounsaturated fats, these good fats help fight bad cholesterol. Polyunsaturated fats stay liquid even in cold temperatures, because their melting point is lower than that of monounsaturated fats. You can find polyunsaturated fats in foods like salmon, fish oil, sunflower oil, and seeds. Polyunsaturated fats contain omega-3 and omega-6 fatty acids, which are often referred to as essential fatty acids (EFAs); these fats are very important. They cannot be manufactured by our bodies, so it is essential to ingest them. This has been made difficult by the fact that omega-3s and omega-6s have largely been processed out of our food chain.

■ **Saturated fat:** Saturated fats might be the most controversial fat you can eat. And with good reason – studies have linked high intake of saturated fats to heart disease. However, those studies have recently been under fire: an updated analysis of many of these studies has revealed that in fact, there was no link at all between fat consumption and rates of heart disease.

Much of the finger-pointing about dietary fat comes from sources like T. Colin Campbell and Thomas Campbell's landmark book *The China Study* and documentaries like *Forks over Knives*, which identified saturated fats and all animal fats as the reasons for nearly all health problems. However, these sources had significant bias toward the saturated fat hypothesis and *completely* ignored populations that had very low incidence of heart disease despite the fact that their diets are rich in saturated fats.

For example, certain hunter-gatherer tribes consume 50 to 70 percent of all their calories from saturated fats without any resulting health problems. In most diets, up to half of the fat consumed may come from saturated fats. And even Walter Willett, chairman of the department of nutrition at Harvard University, reviewed 20 years of research and publicly stated that fats, and more specifically, saturated fats, are not the cause of the obesity crisis or responsible for the incidence of heart disease.

The bottom line is this: saturated fat is one of the best sources of energy for your body. It is why your body *naturally* stores carbohydrates as saturated fat, as research has shown that diets higher in saturated fats are often *lower* in total calories consumed.

■ **Trans fats:** The notable exception. Trans fats, the black sheep of the fat family, are the worst fats. In truth, they are one of the worst forms of food that you could possibly consume. They are found in foods such as French fries, potato chips, and most fried foods. While some trace amounts of trans fats naturally occur in meats and other foods, by and large, most are man-made.

Trans fats are made by a chemical process called partial hydrogenation. To make them, manufacturers pack liquid vegetable oil (an otherwise decent source of monounsaturated fat) with hydrogen atoms, which converts it into a solid fat. As you might imagine, trans fats are ideal for the food industry, because they have a high melting point and a smooth texture, and they can be reused again and again for deep-fat frying.

Essentially, trans fats are a consequence of overprocessing foods in order to offer a longer shelf life. If a food is pre-packaged, it just might contain trans fats. If you are serious about your goals, avoid trans fats at all costs.

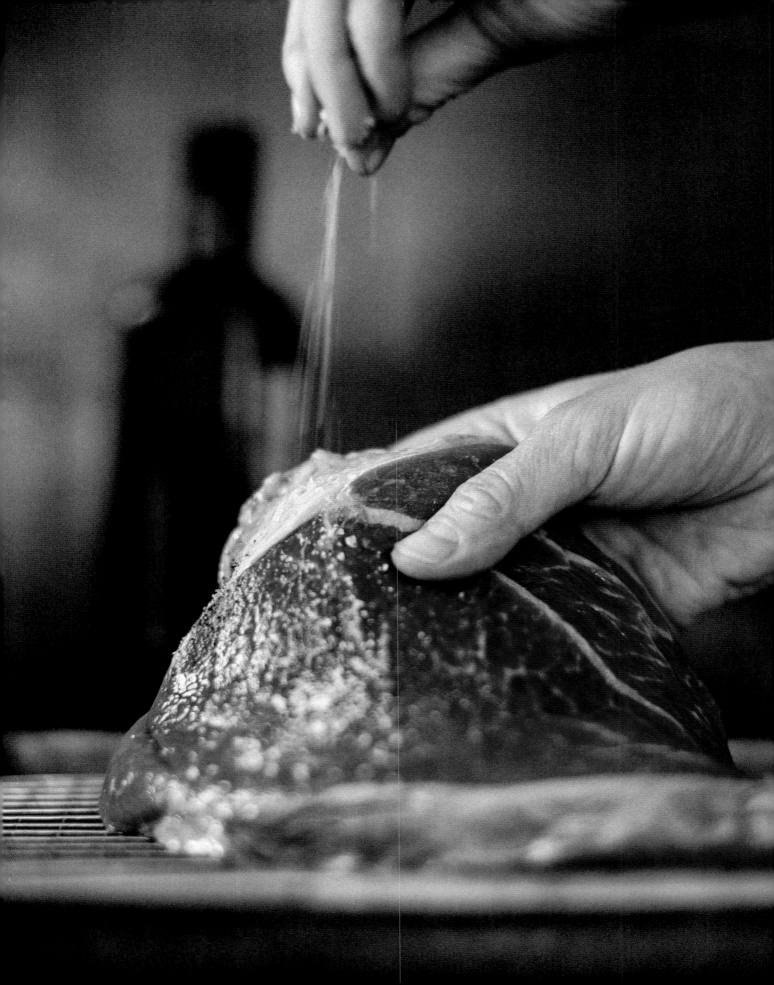

PROTEIN: THE NEW KING?

Protein – we see conflicting information regarding its intake everywhere. Recovery? Protein! Weight loss? Protein! Reduce blood sugar swings? Protein! Body composition change? Protein!

However, there is more to just eating more (or less) protein when it comes to nutrition for athletes. Studies published in peer-reviewed publications point to three primary themes: daily protein intake versus training protein intake; the timing and distribution of protein for strength versus endurance athletes; and protein intake prior to sleep in order to maximize recovery from a muscle and immunity standpoint.

Accrual of skeletal muscle protein requires a sustained positive muscle protein balance (i.e. rates of muscle synthesis exceed muscle breakdown). It is well known that an episode of exercise followed by ingestion of protein helps to stimulate muscle synthesis and maintain a positive nitrogen balance, but there is a gray area: how much protein is necessary? Moreover, what are the critical windows for anabolic stimulus – post-exercise or consumption throughout the day via meals?

The longstanding hypothesis behind post-exercise protein intake has been that ~20 g will provide maximal anabolic stimulus in the early recovery process (~5 hours post exercise). This theory originated in the resistance-training literature and has been generalized to extend to the endurance athlete. However, examination of the endurance literature reveals several other factors that come into play – the athlete's gender, whether the athlete is energy deficient, the composition of the athlete's overall diet (high or low protein), and the composition of the protein the athlete ingests.

Amino Acids and Endurance Exercise

It is well known that carbohydrates are the predominant energy source for continuous endurance events, with fat oxidation playing an increasingly important role in episodes of exercise that extend over 2 hours. However, amino acids from circulation and muscle protein breakdown can provide up to 10% of the total energy during endurance exercise. Amino acids are an excellent source for during higher-intensity, longer-duration exercise, but they are also a good choice when there is low glycogen availability and/or when the athlete follows a habitually high-protein dietary strategy. Although endurance exercise lowers the activity of the enzyme responsible for amino acid use, endurance athletes run the risk of falling into a negative leucine balance. This can thwart the athlete's longer-term goals of muscle mass adaptation and accumulation coupled with body fat mass loss. Thus, amino acids must be replaced through dietary sources.

Amount of Protein

In men, mixed-muscle and myofibrillar protein synthesis rates are enhanced with a small (~10 g) post-exercise ingestion of protein, but further enhanced if the amount of protein increases to ~20 g. Larger amounts (up to 40 g) do not increase synthesis rates, but they do increase amino acid oxidation and urea production.

In women, estrogen inhibits muscle protein synthesis, progesterone enhances muscle breakdown, and a sex difference of hepatic origin exists in amino acid oxidation. With these additional factors, research findings indicate muscle protein synthesis is enhanced with the post-exercise ingestion of ~30 g protein. Here, the leucine content is the contender; muscle protein synthesis is reliance on tissue-leucine concentration; and the effects of estrogen on protein synthesis inhibits the oxidation of leucine within the muscle.

Weight Loss and Lowered Calorie Intake

During either high-intensity training and racing blocks or motivated times of weight loss – or both – a negative energy balance can directly affect recovery, lean mass gain, and subsequent fuel use during training (e.g. greater use of amino acids during exercise). During such periods as these, higher protein intake can greatly benefit lean muscle mass, body fat loss, adaptations, and performance. In fact, the studies Haakonssen et al (2013) and Areta et al (2013) demonstrated a benefit from a daily protein intake of 1.8 to 2.3 g/kg.

The novelty with these studies is not the findings regarding acute post-exercise protein ingestion; instead, it is the finding that ingestion of 4x ~20 g protein over the course of a 12-hour period was shown to elevate muscle protein synthesis. In practical terms, timing protein intake across the day with meals (0.25 g/kg protein per meal) and training can enhance lean mass preservation in times of lowered calorie intake. If dietary changes are made to induce a negative energy balance, protein should not be the main macronutrient excluded.

Types of Protein and Timing of Their Consumption

Dietary proteins differ in their amino acid composition as well as their rates of digestion and absorption. All of these factors have measurable effects on post-exercise muscle protein synthesis and whole-body protein synthesis. The essential amino acid (EAA) content of a protein – in particular, its leucine content – can dramatically affect muscle protein synthesis.

For example, compared with casein and soy sources of protein, whey protein has distinct anabolic characteristics and anti-inflammatory properties that result in greater synthesis of muscle protein. This holds true both at rest and post-exercise. During the overnight fast, casein provided before sleep is absorbed more rapidly than casein provided during the day; in fact, during that period, rates of muscle protein synthesis increased by ~22% as compared to a placebo, and 10% as compared to whey.

Where Does This Leave Me as an Endurance Athlete?

Lean mass and its subsequent function (strength, power, and endurance) are critical to performance, and the support of preservation (during low-energy intake) and adaptation (training stress) is a complex balance.

Ideally, post-exercise ingestion should comprise ~20 to 30 g of high-quality protein within 30 minutes following the exercise. Any delay will compromise tissue leucine concentration and enhance muscle tissue breakdown. There should also be subsequent consumption of ~20 g of protein across the day. Meal content should be ~0.25 g/kg; with one last ingestion of protein before bed. This strategy will support muscle adaptation, body fat loss (with negative energy balance), and lean mass preservation.

SWEET, SWEET SUGAR

What's Sweet on the Tongue Isn't So Sweet in the Body.

With so many different "natural" sweetening agents available today, it is easy to get confused about where each one comes from, its nutritional content, and the different culinary ways to use it. In this book, you will find that the sweeteners of choice include maple syrup, dates, and date syrup. Maple syrup is sweeter on the tongue than sugar (ergo, you use less of it) and is chock full of nutrients. Dates are a very versatile dried fruit that are 100% natural, are unprocessed other than the drying process, and provide a lot of natural fiber, vitamins, and minerals. They are also lower in fructose than most dried fruits.

The following is an explanation of the different sweeteners and sugar substitutes often found in health-oriented cuisine.

Agave Nectar

This syrup comes from the agave cactus plant. Unfortunately, Hollywood and the media have glorified this sweetener as a raw, natural sweetener with health benefits. In reality, agave is actually a less healthy choice, and even *more* harmful than high-fructose corn syrup. Agave has an unbelievably high amount of fructose and is not natural or raw in *any* form - even if the bottle claims that it's raw.

Agave is mostly fructose, which of course is a natural source of sugar. However, the fructose that occurs naturally is found in minimal amounts in fruits and some vegetables, and in those fruits and vegetables, it is balanced out with fiber and other nutrients. So in its natural state, fructose is great.

However, agave is actually anywhere from 70% to 90% fructose — way more than nature intended and way more than our bodies can handle. It is very difficult for the body to regulate this amount of fructose at once; as such, agave can have damaging effects on your metabolism, memory, concentration, and of course, weight.

Honey

Likely the world's oldest natural sweetener, honey's flavor and color varies significantly depending on what flower's nectar was used by the bees to make it. It is about twice as sweet as regular table sugar and contains several trace minerals and B vitamins. One tablespoon has 64 calories and 17.3 g of sugar.

Maple Syrup

Pure maple syrup is extracted directly from a plant source. It is extracted by tapping maple trees; the sap in the bark leaks out, is collected, and is boiled down until a syrup is formed. Maple syrup is rich in manganese, thiamine (B1), and zinc, and it contains polyphenols with anti-inflammatory properties. Altogether, maple syrup has more than 54 antioxidants that help fight free radicals and give your immune system a major boost. The benefits of maple syrup rival that of fresh, raw berries; tomatoes; flax seeds; and tea.

Molasses

There are several different types of molasses, each with a different flavor profile and culinary use. Molasses is the material left over in sugar production after the juice of sugar beets or sugar canes is extracted, boiled, and crystallized.

Molasses is about 65% as sweet as table sugar. When possible, opt for unsulfured molasses. One tablespoon of molasses contains 58 calories and 15 g of sugar. The three different types of molasses are:

- **Light molasses:** The syrup leftover after the beets or cane are boiled the first time.

- **Dark molasses:** The syrup leftover after the beets or cane are boiled the second time.

- **Blackstrap molasses:** The thick, dark molasses leftover after sugar beets or cane is refined into table sugar in its third boiling. Its flavor is best described as bittersweet; blackstrap works well in chilis, baked beans, cookies, and roasted chicken or turkey. A sweet note: this type of molasses contains calcium, iron, copper, potassium, magnesium, manganese, selenium, and vitamin B6.

Per 60 ml portion in %DV[1]	Maple syrup of Canada	Honey	Sugar	Brown sugar	Agave syrup
Manganese	100 *	3	0	9 #	0
Riboflavin (B$_2$)	37 *	2	1	0	0
Zinc	18 **	2	0	1	0
Magnesium	7 #	1	0	7 #	0
Calcium	5 #	0	0	5 #	0
Potassium	5 #	1	0	6 #	0
Calories	217	261	196	211	256
Sugars (in G)	54	72	51	54	56

* Excellent source of   /   ** Good source of   /   # Source of

[1]**DV:** The *Daily Value* is the amount deemed sufficient to meet the daily needs of the majority of healthy individuals.
Source: Canadian Nutrient File (Health Canada)

SUGAR SUBSTITUTES: NOT A HEALTHY CHOICE

Sugar substitutes, which are often known as artificial sweeteners, have come into the spotlight recently due to evidence that they affect the gut microbiome (the bacteria in your gut) and promote obesity and glucose intolerance. In humans, the ability to digest and extract energy from food is determined not only by our genes but also by the activity of the trillions of microbes that dwell within our digestive tracts; collectively, these bacteria are known as the gut microbiome. Recent research has revealed that artificial sweeteners enhance the populations of gut bacteria that are more efficient at pulling energy from food and turning that energy into fat.

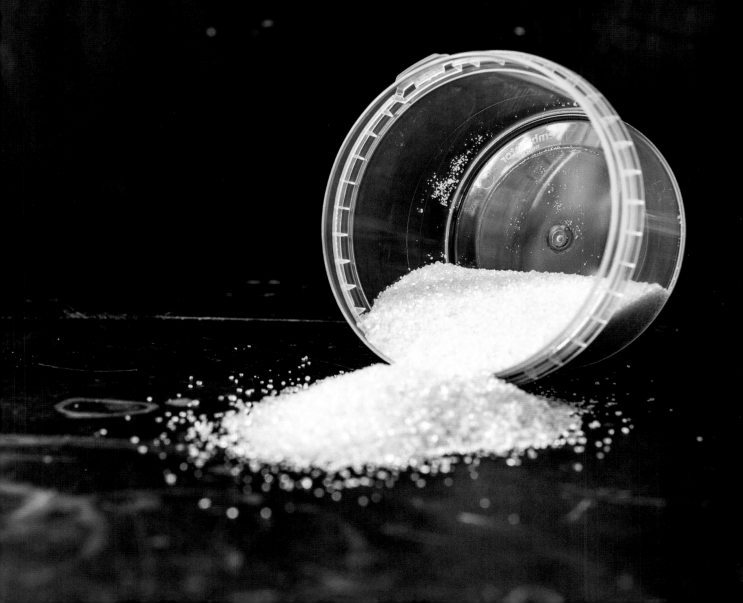

A brief background on the gut microbiome: contrary to popular belief, the microorganisms hosted by a human body aren't really working *for us*. They are interested in their own survival and reproduction, but they cannot survive on their own. So, by design, they have a symbiotic relationship with their human host.

The relationship can be beneficial to both parties, but this is not always the case. For example, there are microorganisms in your gut that ferment polysaccharides (chains of sugar) into energy for you to use, which is a positive byproduct of their activity. Others expend their energy fighting one another, suppressing the growth of other microorganisms to optimize their own living conditions. Sometimes this is to your benefit, as in the case of a species called bifidobacterium. This bacteria alters the gut environment in positive ways at the expense of not-so-beneficial bacteria.

However, other microbial turf wars can be detrimental to human health. Your gut bacteria also assist in the production of hormones, the regulation of immunity, and even the manipulation of your moods, which is especially noticeable when you are lacking certain key microbes. For example, as levels of important gut flora, such as the *Lactobacilli* strain (part of the *Firmicutes* variety) decline, various symptoms of psychological distress increase, including anxiety, poor sleep, and heart rate. On the flip side, research shows that mood significantly improves when healthy levels of these bacteria are restored.

Another important finding was that the proportion of *Bacteroidetes* to *Firmicutes* bacteria levels increase as people lose weight through either a low-fat or low-carbohydrate diet. These findings suggest that the bacteria in the human gut may not only influence our ability to extract calories and store energy from our diet; they may also affect the balance of hormones, such as leptin, that shape our eating behavior, leading some of us to eat more than others.

During Exercise

Different types of artificial sweeteners consumed during exercise can bring on changes in osmotic and oncotic pressures, which can pull water out of the blood and into the GI tract. For example, the sugar alcohols sorbitol mannitol and xylitol are commonly used as laxatives because they pull water into the intestines. The sweetener sucralose induces an insulin spike – rather, your body perceives that sweetness is being consumed and in response releases insulin to combat the anticipated sugar. When none does, your existing blood glucose gets taken up into the body. The drop in blood glucose causes a bit of hypoglycemia, signaling your body to release more glucose into the blood, which causes insulin to be released around and around it goes.

If consumed during exercise, products containing sucralose will make your blood sugar "bottom out" (kind of like taking in lots of caffeine) and increase your carbohydrate requirements. Sucralose is also linked to GI distress symptoms, including diarrhea, bloating, and gas.

BEVERAGES

The composition (as well as the concentration) of the fluids you consume while exercising is important. For optimum hydration, your body relies on fluid cotransporters, which are essentially molecular pilots that carry fluid across your intestinal cells and into the water spaces of the body.

Sodium, a Top Gun-level pilot for hydration, works best when it has a good co-pilot, and glucose is its co-pilot of choice. Sodium can be absorbed into your cells by a few different mechanisms, but mostly, it hitches a ride with glucose. Without glucose, the constant flow of sodium and water into your bloodstream slows. This is why sports drinks that actually do hydrate and do not just sit in the stomach and cause sloshing, bloating, and discomfort contain a small amount of sugar (glucose and sucrose) as well as sodium to optimize their absorption and hydration.

Avoid typical sports drinks, as they are too concentrated in carbohydrates to properly hydrate. The first purpose of these drinks is to supply carbohydrates for fuel. Instead, seek out a sports drink that supplies glucose, sodium, and other key cotransporters as described above. A winning drink contains the following per 250mL:

- Carbohydrate solution: 3% to 4%
  (7-9.4 g carb per 250 mL)

- Sugars: 7 to 9.4 g from glucose and sucrose

- Sodium: 180 to 225 mg

- Potassium (another fluid co-transporter):
  60 to 75 mg

You can make this simple solution at home: 1/16th of a teaspoon of salt (250 mg sodium), 1 teaspoon of maple syrup (5 g carbohydrate), and the juice of 1 lemon (3 g carb, 60 mg potassium). During the day, stay hydrated by drinking fluids and consuming watery fruits and veggies with a sprinkle of salt. Rely on the salt/ maple/ date syrup/ lemon juice solution to ensure total hydration.

For fuel and recovery foods, refer to the following chart:

	Good	Okay	Not Good
Night before a morning event or morning of an afternoon event	Waffles / whole grain pancakes and bread / oatmeal / quinoa / fish / poultry / salad (be careful with fiber)	Real food that you normally have for dinner or breakfast	High-fat, high-protein meal (no more than 20 g to 25 g of protein) / anything fructose-based
1-3 hours before	Bananas / grapes / oranges / berries / bircher muesli / toast with almond or other nut butter	Sandwich	Dairy / apples / grapefruit
0-1 hour before	10 g to 15 g of protein 30 minutes before heading out / fat-free unsweetened yogurt / almond butter and jam sandwich on low-fiber bread / almond milk with a bit of whey protein powder	Low-fiber toast and jam / English muffin with a low-fat spread / small handful of nuts and a banana	Anything fructose-based / anything high-fat or high-protein
During	40 g to 50 g of carbs per hour of exercise / salted new potatoes / sandwich bites / low-fat muffin / pretzel bites / jelly beans or Swedish fish	Uncoated protein bar (190–210 calories, 6 g to 10 g protein) / exercise-specific blocks / trail mix, depending on the intensity of exercise	Fruit-based bars (too high in fructose) / Gatorade and other 5–8%-carbohydrate drinks / gels and GUs
After / recovery	Restock protein within 30 minutes 25 g to 30 g animal protein / 20 g to 25 g whey-casein combination Restock carbs within 90 minutes (sources rich in glucose are ideal) PB&J or turkey and cheese sandwich / any type of lean protein—chicken breast, fish, etc. / starchy veggies, such as potatoes, peas, and corn / root veggies, such as parsnips / smoothie of frozen banana or mango with whey protein powder and fat-free Greek yogurt and almond milk	Wraps (veggie, lean protein, hummus) / small bean and rice burrito with salsa (no guacamole or sour cream) / low-fat or fat-free mocha with low-fat muffin or bagel with low-fat spread	Any processed sugar, candy, or engineered nutrition — the only exception is protein powder, which can be either whey isolate, casein isolate, quinoa, or hemp — no soy!

The way to anyone's general health and physical performance is through his or her stomach — more specifically, the gut. In fact, the bacteria that live in your digestive tract influence pretty much everything in your body, so it is absolutely crucial to take care of your gut. Your gut bacteria assist in the production of hormones and regulation of the immune system, and they even manipulate your moods, especially when you are lacking certain key microbes.

For example, as levels of certain important gut flora, such as the Lactobacilli strain (part of the Firmicutes variety) decline, various symptoms of psychological distress increase. On the flip side, research shows that mood significantly improves when healthy levels of these bacteria are restored. If you choose to starve your important flora through fasting, you will effectively limit the nutrients these bacteria need to grow and thrive. As a result, your pain perception will increase as your gut sends the message that you are not able to work hard until you get the nourishment you need.

The easiest way to manipulate your gut flora is by enriching your diet with a variety of probiotics and prebiotics. Probiotics are the actual bacteria that live in your gut, and prebiotics are the substances the bacteria eat. Food sources are the best way to get both of these, since the diversity of the bacteria in supplements is not as varied as they are in nature; a second choice could be a high-quality, supplement rich in specific flora.

The first step is to eat a balanced diet rich in variety. Individual microbes flourish when they are exposed to different foods and nutrients. If your diet is out of balance, your gut bacteria will be too. This sets up a vicious and unhealthy cycle in which one type of bacteria dominates over others.

By balancing your diet, you can break this cycle and establish a rich, diverse colony of gut bacteria that includes the varieties associated with leanness and health. Studies have shown that lean people have a richer, more diverse gut colony than obese people. The most essential dietary component for all beneficial bacteria is fiber, so get at least 25 grams a day from a wide variety of foods, especially vegetables and legumes.

The next step is to make sure that your daily diet is rich in specific probiotics. Probiotics come in many different forms, including such fermented foods as kimchi, sauerkraut, soft and aged cheeses, miso paste, sourdough bread, and probiotic heavy hitters like kefir and yogurt. Probiotic foods establish a healthy colony of microbes in your gut, which in turn send messages to the brain via the vagus nerve that everything is OK in the intestines, so calm down and stop craving sweets!

Of course, probiotics also aid with digestion, which in and of itself can yield dramatic benefits. In one particularly revealing study, a group of overweight women and men kept their calories constant but changed their diet to include a probiotic-rich yogurt. They did not eat less or exercise more, but after just six weeks on the diet, participants lost an average of 4 percent of their body fat. This was achieved simply by improving their digestive health, which in turn boosted their metabolism and led to fat loss and healthier body composition.

Simple Hydration Drink

500 ml water
1 tbsp. maple syrup
½ lemon, juice
1/16 tsp. salt

Mix all the ingredients together and cool down.

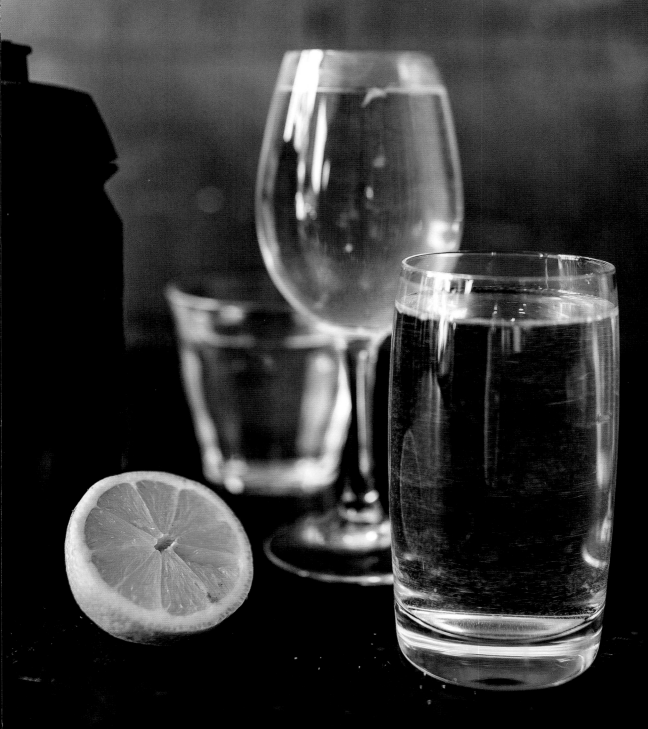

JET LAG

Jet lag means a temporary disruption of normal circadian rhythm caused by high-speed travel across several time zones typically in a jet aircraft, resulting in fatigue, disorientation, and disturbed sleep patterns.

With the globalization of racing and the relative ease of travel, it is hard not to pick a destination race or even fly from the east to west coast. However, the dreaded time-lag toll on the body can seriously hinder how we feel and perform! The swollen ankles and dead legs over the first few hours of the day after a long-haul flight, not to mention the extreme waves of tiredness and lethargy, affect so many things, so how do we as athletes thwart the dreaded jet lag so we can race well and enjoy the trip?

Jet lag itself is different from travel fatigue. Travel fatigue can usually be solved by a good meal, rehydration, and a great sleep. Jet lag, on the other hand, is caused by a temporary misalignment between our internal body clock controlling our circadian rhythms and the destination time zone and sleep/wake cycle. It is interesting to note that it takes longer to reset the circadian clock following an eastward than a westward flight (primarily because the human circadian clock is slightly longer than 24 hours); so we have a natural tendency to drift slightly later each day.

Why pay so much attention to the body clock? Generally, feeling tired is part of what we experience as an athlete and it is generally accepted that sleep loss has minimal effect on muscle strength; but a significant contribution to the "on-fire" performance we want in a race is the trained nuances of our body clock. Our core temperature, hormone production, and plasma concentrations of melatonin all play a role in achieving top performance.

What to do?

The best way to alleviate jetlag is to adjust the body clock. The biggest contributors to lingering jet lag are the changes in the light-dark cycle, night time melatonin production, and exercise (core temperature fluctuations). It is pretty unlikely that we have the luxury of changing our sleep-wake cycles before we leave to match our destination, but there are a few things you can do before leaving that will help upon arrival.

Exposure to bright light coupled with melatonin production: Melatonin production lowers core temperature, and the onset of sleep requires a vasodilation with a drop in core temperature. Think about a hot night when you cannot sleep because you are too hot, so you get up and drink cold water or stick your feet out from under the covers. This helps to dissipate heat and allows your core temperature to drop; so sleep ensues!

For flying east: To start the reset process, for four days before your trip, drink ~100mL COLD tart cherry juice 30 minutes before bedtime. Go to bed 1 hour earlier, and get up 1 hour earlier than usual. When you wake, get bright light exposure as soon as possible (preferably by going outside, but a bright SAD light or similar light will work too). Just one or two days of a preflight sleep-shift will help reduce subsequent jet lag.

For flying west: Since flying west is easier for adjusting the circadian rhythms due to the body's natural tendency for a longer day, delaying bedtime is effective at resetting the body clock. Remember, the more time zones you cross, the bigger the jet lag effect. With this in mind, delaying your bedtime by an hour a night for the 2-4 nights before your flight will help. This is not really that practical for our normal busy schedules, as ideally, you would want to wake up an hour later. If you can sleep an extra 30-60 minutes and expose yourself to bright light first thing when you wake up, it will help.

What about the days before and on the actual day of travel?

Flying long distances, especially through several time zones, is very stressful for the body. The plane's environment will probably be lower in oxygen than the regular atmosphere and also quite dry, which may cause you to become dehydrated. Travellers who drink alcoholic beverages will experience worse dehydration problems.

Tips

The week before your trip, load up immune and gut boosting foods (you may consider taking something like Good Gut Daily Boost), and take one 80 mg aspirin per day (as a pre-emptive for deep vein thrombosis).

Food over the four days preceding your flight:

DAY 1	Eat a high-protein breakfast and lunch but a high-carbohydrate, low-protein dinner.
DAY 2	Eat light meals of salads, thin soups / smoothies, fruits, juices, veggies; keeping fats and calories at a minimum (kind of like a moderate fast).
DAY 3	Repeat Day 1.
Day 4 (Flight)	Departure Day: Repeat Day 2 (Compression tights are magic!)

Flying Eastward	On the day of travel, consume caffeinated beverages only between your normal hours of 6–11 a.m. If you are landing at your destination at night, then sleeping on the plane is not a great idea. Try to stay awake.
Flying Westward	On the day of travel, drink caffeinated drinks only in the morning of your usual time. If you are landing at your destination in the morning / daytime, then drinking tart cherry juice or taking valerian capsules will help you sleep on the plane without waking up feeling 'hungover'.

Avoid caffeine and alcohol as they will make you dehydrated. Every 2-3 hours during your flight, drink 500-800 mL functional hydration (i.e. add 1/16th tsp. of salt into that 500-800 mL) plus 80 mg aspirin. This combination will help with dehydration and prevent DVTs.

Have a protein drink (e.g. take protein powder onto your flight and mix it with juice or water) for every 6 hours of flying: this helps to keep you hydrated, and reduces hunger.

- Do not forget to get up every 90-120 minutes (if you are not sleeping) and walk around OR do some isometric exercises in your seat to keep the blood flowing!

- Upon landing, have another protein drink; again for rehydration and light fueling.

- If you land during the day, go outside without sunglasses to use sunlight to reset your body clock. This will help you adjust to the new time zone.

- If time allows, get out for a walk or easy spin to bring your heart rate up and help alleviate any swelling. Running will be more damaging after a long haul flight of sitting, due to the sudden impact on the muscles. All lower body compartments will be a bit swollen, so walking is the primary, least damaging way to reset the fluid shifts. A light spin or a swim is also great, but you will want to be exposed to bright light if you land in the day, so take that into consideration as well.

- A high-carbohydrate, low-fat and low-sugar meal will make it easier to sleep either on the plane or at your destination. However, if you need to be alert, eat a high-protein but low in fat and sugar diet.

- A high-protein meal will increase alertness and ability to think clearly. Have a low-carbohydrate, high protein-breakfast either on the plane or upon landing if you are landing and need to stay awake!

The high-protein meals, exercises and light are intended to stimulate the body's active cycle. The high-carbohydrate meals stimulate sleep. Caffeine and its chemical relatives can cause your biological rhythms to shift forward or backward, depending on the time they are consumed. Between 3 and 5 p.m., their effect is neutral.

Although transmeridian travel is becoming essential, the subsequent jet lag is not a necessary evil. Doing things to reset your circadian rhythms before you go and upon landing is kind of like packing your bike box - a pain at times, but well worth it!

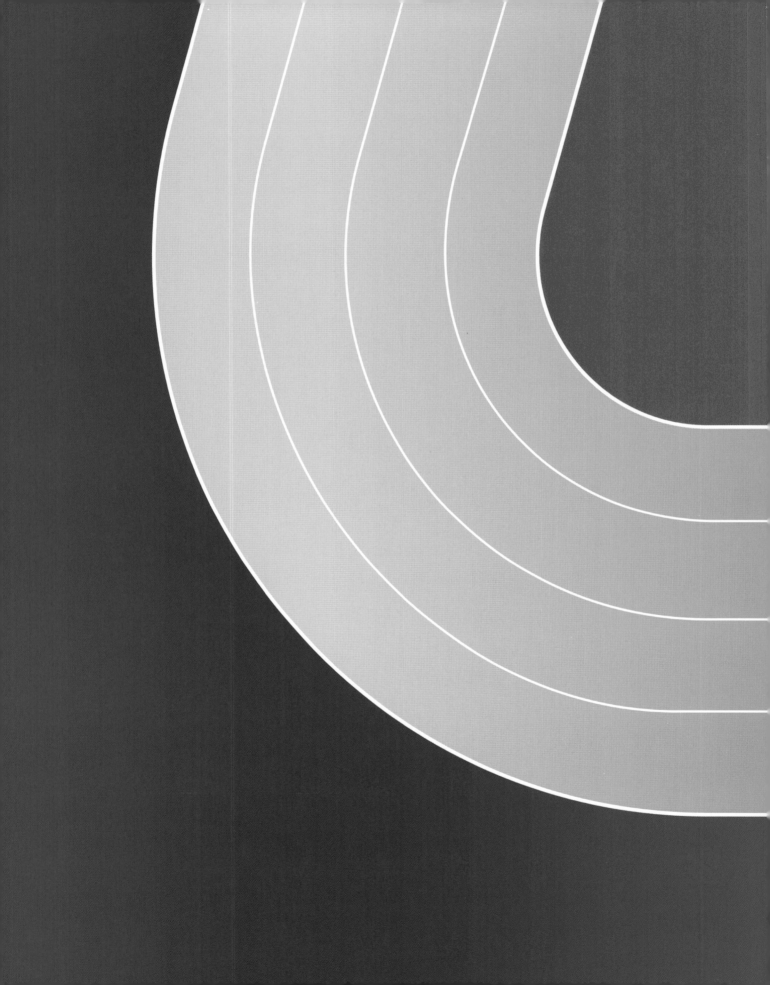

WINTER
ERW TER

Winter Breakfasts

Winter Lunches, Dinners and Sides

WINTER: PRE-SEASON

In winter, the days draw to a close early and temperatures drop. Less-than-ideal weather conditions mean most of us turn to indoor training by way of cycling classes, ergometers, treadmills, indoor pools, and the like. While none of these choices are overly inspiring, they keep us fit so that when the real work begins, we are not starting from nothing!

Due to the shorter days and cooler temperatures, our metabolism changes to promote increased fat storage and the use of carbohydrates throughout the day. We also tend to crave more nutrient-dense foods and warmth. As such, a diet that is lower in carbohydrates and higher in fats and protein is well-suited to winter. The recipes in this section have been created to increase satiation, reduce calorie intake, as well as increase lean mass preservation, immunity, and sleep quality.

Eat Race Win! Keywords for Winter

- Reduced carbohydrate intake
- Increased protein intake (i.e. fish, eggs, duck, beef, pork)
- Increased intake of low-sugar fruits and root vegetables
- Maple/date syrup
- Quinoa, beans, lentils, amaranth, and sweet potatoes
- Skyr, 2% fat milk, yogurt, cream, cheeses, and almond milk
- Probiotics for the gut microbiome to improve the immune system, reduce stress, and increase the quality of sleep
- Fats, including olive and rice bran oils
- Nuts and seeds
- Vinaigrettes and low-fat sauces
- No foods high in sugars

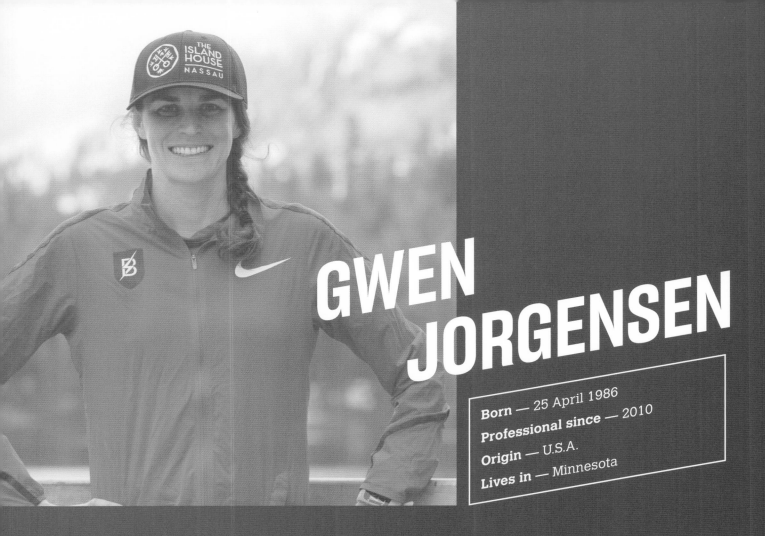

GWEN JORGENSEN

Born — 25 April 1986
Professional since — 2010
Origin — U.S.A.
Lives in — Minnesota

It's easier to ask Gwen Jorgensen what she hasn't won. In her career, she's been a national, world, and Olympic champion, as well as a two-time winner of U.S.A. Triathlon's Triathlete of the Year. She attributes a huge part of her success to nutrition and diet. "The importance of food is enormous," she says. "Nutrition is so important for better recovery and more energy." She eats plenty of whole foods, and has worked on increasing her calorie intake through avocados, oils, nuts, and coconut: "Three years ago, I lost a lot of weight and worked on adding fats into my diet rather than carbs."

Food for triathletes is "a very personal thing," Gwen shares. "Nutrition is as important as training." She works with a nutritionist who regularly does blood tests to check on vital statistics like her iron levels (she eats a lot of morcilla to keep them up) and has altered her diet by frontloading her day with smoothies, bananas, and peanut butter for extra calories. "I feel better if I know I eat well," she says. "When I eat healthily, I know I'm doing everything I can to recover right and build performance confidence." Gwen also feels that she performs better when she eliminates gluten, and estimates that 90% of her food shopping is gluten-free: "Bread in the U.S.A. can be bad, but fresh sourdough bread makes me feel so much better."

Gwen prefers to keep her diet natural and does not use engineered nutrition like gels, as "they make your teeth rot," she says. "Train on what you're going to have on race day. Foods like bananas are for training, and not for racing." She mentions that 400 kcal is enough to sustain her efforts. And for recovery? "I use nutritional bars or send my husband out for food." She's a great believer in eating local cuisine "to experience the place and culture, whether that's meat pies in Wellington or paella in Valencia." When she's not doing so, her favorite meals during the season are rice dishes and sweet potato salads: "Sweet potatoes are an absolute favorite of mine, so you'll almost always find them on my plate for dinner!"

Gwen is married to former pro cyclist Patrick Lemieux, who knows exactly what it takes to be an elite athlete. Describing himself as her house-husband, it's Patrick who shops and cooks for Gwen so that she can focus on her training. "I eat a lot, and my day typically has 3-4 training passes so I try to pack in a lot of calories in the morning to have a base of energy to take from. I've found that if I lay low on breakfast, I don't perform as well as on the days when I eat a proper, solid breakfast." So how does a champion triathlete start the day? "A typical breakfast for me would be oatmeal with a variation of nuts and seasonal fruits, plus a poached egg for protein. It lasts me a long time and is easy to make wherever we are in the world."

For lunch, she prefers rice-based meals, cooked vegetables, and some sort of protein. "Some of my favorite lunch and post-race style dishes would be rice curries and pad thai. They are easy to eat and palatable." As she usually frontloads her nutrition, dinner is always the lightest meal of the day with plenty of cooked vegetables: "I ALWAYS eat something green with my meals." On lighter training days, she keeps it super-simple with a frittata, and when she's traveling, Patrick can be relied upon to make her something suitable for the flights.

Knowing what to fuel up on during a training ride can be tricky, but Gwen keeps it fuss-free: a water bottle full of Red Bull diluted 50/50 with water, bananas, as well as organic and natural nutrition bars: "I always check the ingredients." On an important race day, she'll eat a bowl of oats soaked overnight with peanut butter about 3½ hours prior to the start. If she's racing later in the day, then it'll be rice and yogurt for breakfast plus oats and a nutrition bar. Does she take the temperature into consideration when she's planning her race nutrition? "That's definitely something I consider. On a cold day, it takes around 2½ hours to digest a pre-race meal, but on a hot day, I give myself longer. Hydration is essential for hot days, so I make sure to take on enough fluids. For example, I freeze my water bottles and let them thaw so that the water ends up cool, but not icy."

Has she noticed a change in the way triathletes eat over the last couple of years? She echoes the advice of other endurance athletes: "Don't try anything crazy. Stick to what works and what doesn't work for you." Her best advice for newcomers to the sport is to frontload daily nutrition with go-to recipes that allow them to plan without having to struggle to find things to eat. "Plan food, cook ahead, and have the right foods available." She also shares that not eating enough is a rookie mistake she knows from her own experience of "waking up at 2 a.m. after a race, starving, and eating ice cream! Eating enough at the right times will also help you to avoid empty calories."

So what does Gwen Jorgensen, one of the world's top performers, consider her greatest victory? "It's not just about finishing first. It's about what you've accomplished and how you've grown as a person; pushing your own boundaries. The experiences you have along the way with family, food, and travels are all a part of that - so don't take them for granted."

"Nutrition is so important for better recovery and more energy. [It] is as important as training."

Kasha and Poached Eggs with Arugula

To prepare the buckwheat: In a medium-sized pot over medium heat, combine the buckwheat, salted water and garlic, then bring them to a boil. Reduce the heat to low and simmer covered for 10–12 minutes until all the liquid has been absorbed. Remove it from the heat and set it aside to rest covered for 10 minutes. Uncover, mash the soft garlic with a fork, and stir until well combined.

———

To prepare the eggs: Bring 2 medium-sized pots of salted water to a boil over medium heat. Crack the eggs into 2 separate small bowls and remove any pieces of shell. With 1 hand, place 4 fingers like a claw over the first egg and carefully tilt the bowl so that the thinnest part of the egg white drains into the sink. Repeat this with the second egg. Add the white wine vinegar to the first pot and swirl the water around with a whisk in a sturdy pace, creating a vortex in the center. Drop the first egg into the center of the vortex and let the water spin around the egg. The egg white should set into a beautiful sphere. Once it has set, cook until it is stable enough to be lifted out of the pot with a slotted spoon. Transfer it into the second pot and poach to the desired level of doneness (for a soft, runny yolk: 4 minutes/for a soft, firm yolk: 4–5 minutes/for a set yolk: 5 minutes – cooking times vary depending on the eggs' size and freshness). Repeat this process with the second egg.

———

In a small bowl, whisk the olive oil and the apple cider vinegar together. Add the arugula and flip it around until it is well coated. Season with salt and pepper to taste. Serve by distributing the warm buckwheat into 2 bowls, then topping each of them with a handful of arugula and a poached egg.

200 g buckwheat (kasha), rinsed in cold water

200 mL water with 1 tsp. salt + more as needed

2 cloves garlic, peeled

2 whole large eggs

50 mL white wine vinegar

1 tbsp. olive oil

Apple cider vinegar, to taste

1 handful (20 g) fresh arugula, rinsed and dried

Salt and pepper, to taste

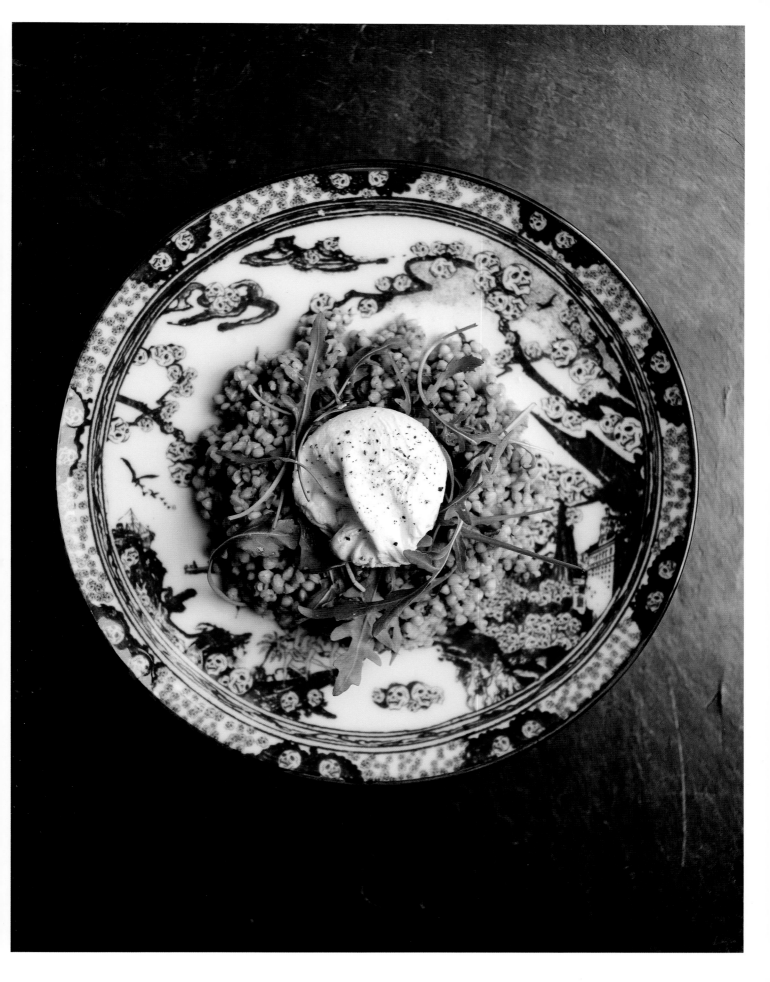

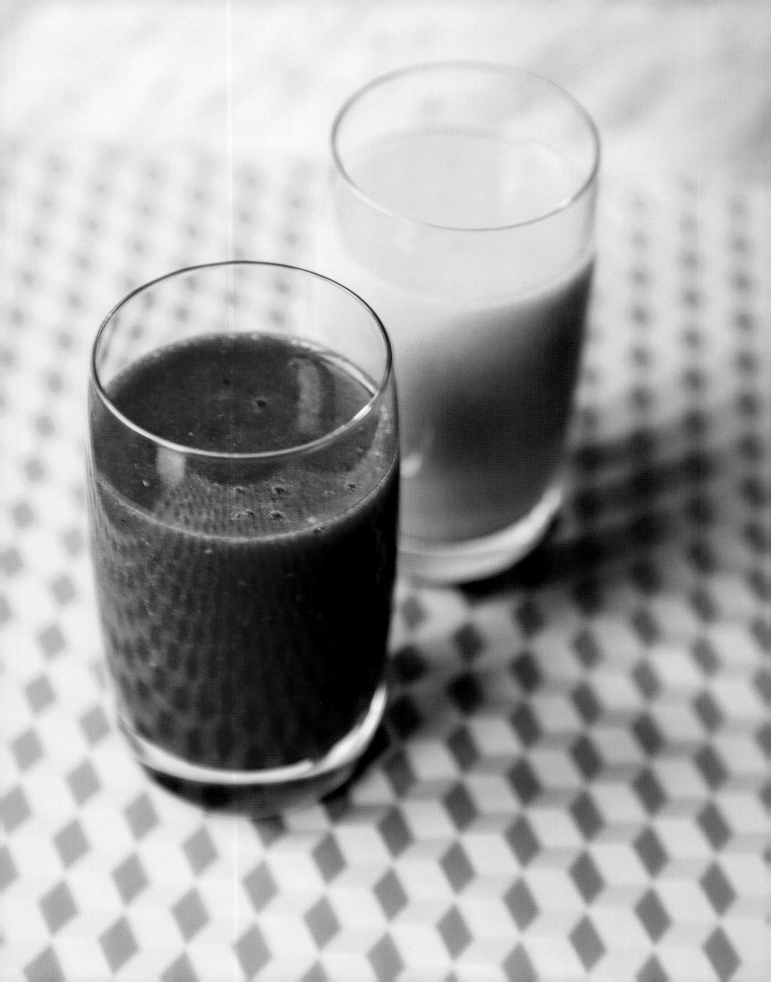

Mango-oat Smoothie with Ginger and Lime

G D N V

Slice the mango on each side of its stone and scoop the flesh out. In the jug of a powerful blender, combine the mango flesh, banana, oatmeal and ½ of the carrot juice. Blend until smooth. Add the ginger and blend again until smooth. Add the remaining juice and water if needed, then blend again until the desired consistency. Season with lime zest and juice to taste, then serve.

1 medium mango

1 medium banana, peeled

100 g cold cooked oatmeal (porridge)

250 mL carrot juice, divided

20 g fresh ginger, peeled and thinly sliced

Zest and juice of 1 lime, to taste

Beet and Raspberry Smoothie

Re G D N V

In the jug of a powerful blender, combine the beet juice, banana and raspberries. Blend until smooth. Add water if needed, then blend again until the desired consistency. Season with honey, lime zest and juice to taste, then serve.

TIP: Make it thinner and drink it on-the-go, or serve it thicker in a bowl with müesli and a scoop of Greek yogurt. Add protein powder to promote recovery.

250 mL beet juice

1 medium banana, peeled

150 g frozen raspberries

Honey, to taste

Zest and juice of 1 lime, to taste

Go Away, Cold!
Golden Root Oatmeal

G D V

In a large pot over medium heat, combine the water, raisins, sunflower seeds, dried apples, spices and salt, then bring them to a boil. While stirring constantly, add the oats and return them to a boil. Add ½ of the diced apples, then reduce the heat to low and simmer for 10 minutes. Add water if needed, then season with salt and honey to taste.

—

Transfer the oatmeal into serving bowls and top each serving with sunflower seeds, the remaining diced apples and honey to taste, then serve.

1 L water + more as needed

50 g golden sultana raisins

20 g sunflower seeds + more to serve

15 g dried apples

1 tsp. freshly grated ginger pulp or ¼ tsp. dry ginger

1 tsp. freshly grated turmeric root or ¼ tsp. turmeric powder

½ tsp. ground cinnamon

Salt, to taste

200 g rolled oats

2 medium apples, diced and divided

Honey, maple or date syrup, to taste

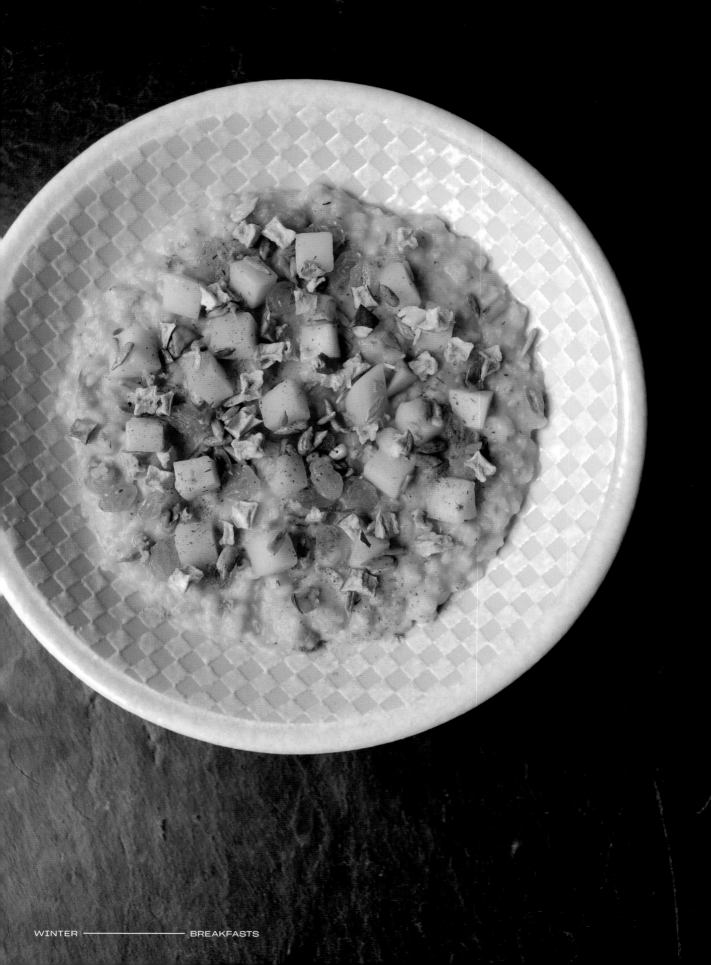

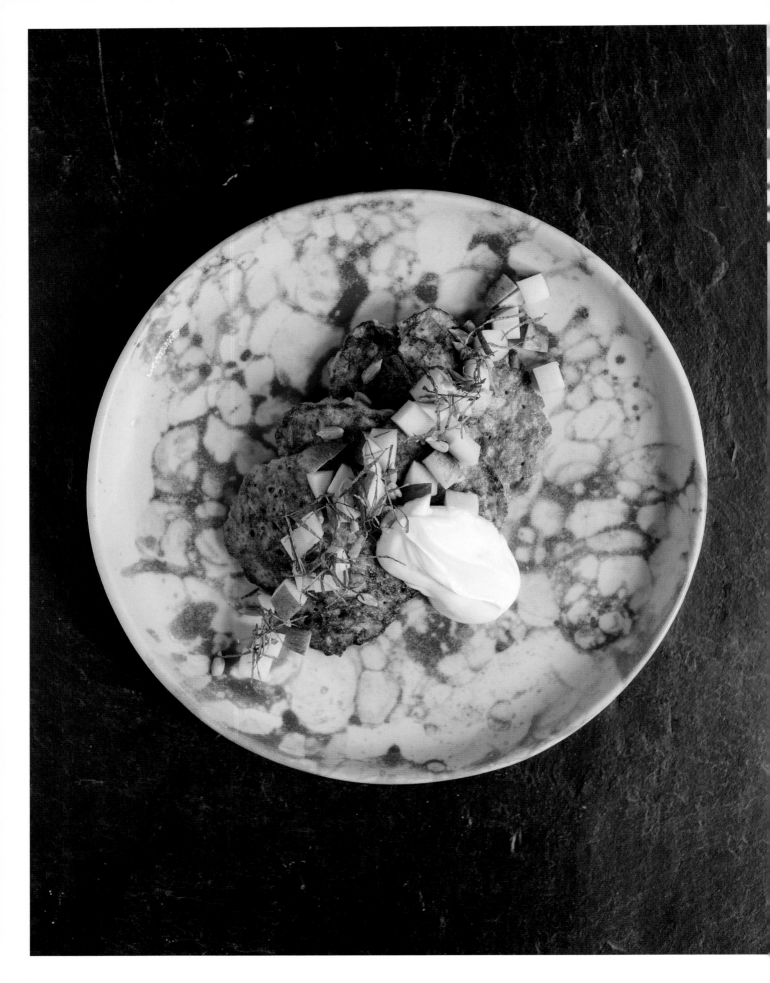

Golden Fried Porridge Pancakes

Whisk the eggs into the porridge until smooth. Heat up a non-stick pan with ½ tbsp. of olive oil. Add 3 spoons of porridge onto the pan and fry for 2 minutes on each side until golden and firm.
Transfer the fried porridge pancakes onto plates. Top with fresh fruit, yogurt and honey to your liking, then serve.

2 eggs

200 g leftover oatmeal (porridge)

Olive oil, to fry

1 pinch salt

Fresh fruit, to serve

Yogurt, to serve

Honey, to serve

Egg Wraps with Banana, Pineapple, Almond Butter, and Lime

ii

2 whole large eggs

1 pinch ground cinnamon

Salt, to taste

1 banana, peeled and sliced

100 g fresh pineapple, diced

1 passion fruit

15 mL honey, or to taste

Zest and juice of 1 lime

1 tsp. olive oil

30 g almond butter

Plain Greek yogurt, to serve

Ⓖ Ⓓ Ⓥ

In a small mixing bowl, whisk the eggs and cinnamon together, then season with salt to taste. Set it aside. In another mixing bowl, combine the banana, pineapple and passion fruit seeds. Gently mix them together, then season with honey, lime zest and juice to taste.

—

In a non-stick pan over medium heat, heat up the oil. Pour ½ of the egg mixture into the pan, then spread it thinly and evenly into a pancake form. Cook for about 45 seconds. Flip it over and cook for another 15 seconds, until the pancake sets completely. Transfer it onto a serving plate. Repeat this process with the remaining egg mixture. Spread the almond butter on each pancake, top them with ½ of the fruit salad each, then roll them up. Serve with yogurt and honey to taste.

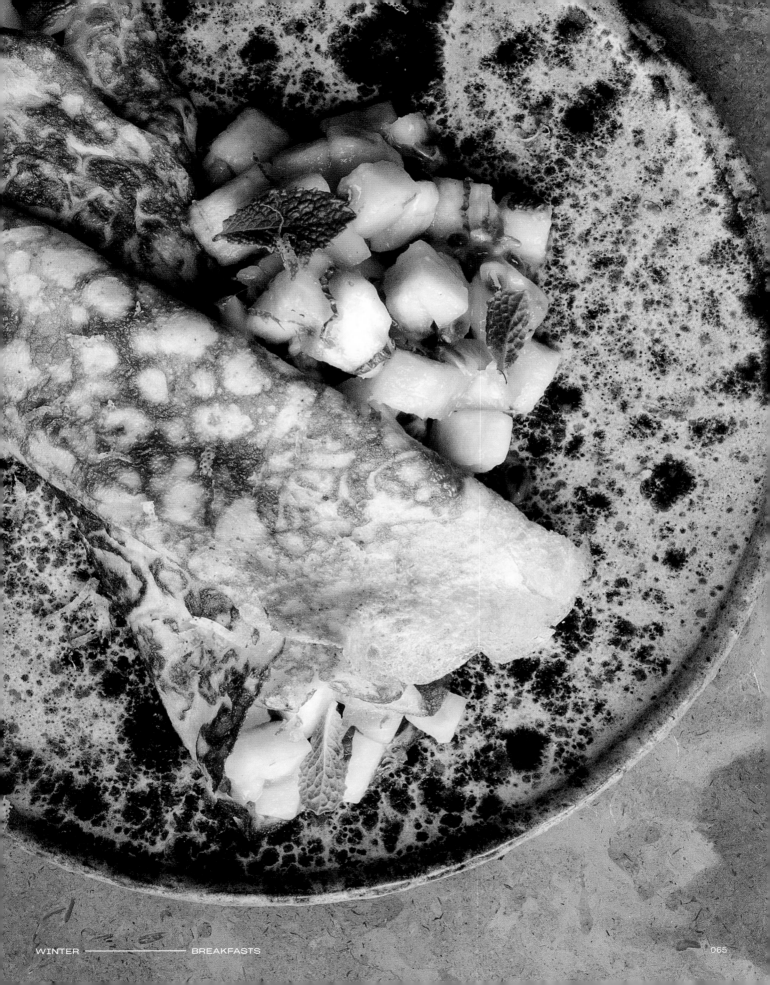

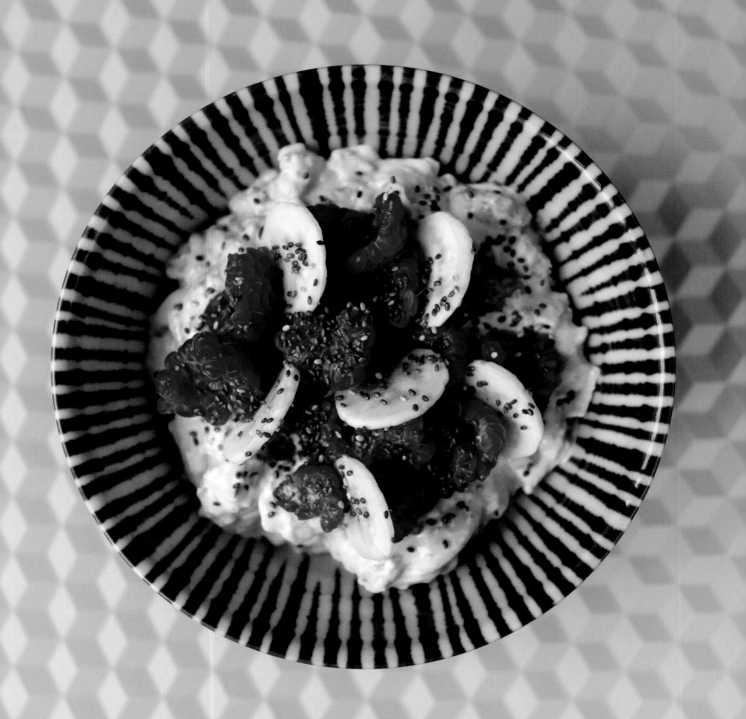

Bircher Müesli with Chia, Banana, and Raspberry

In a mixing bowl, combine the müesli, yogurt, chia seeds and banana. Cover it with plastic wrap and refrigerate overnight. Remove the plastic wrap and stir the mixture well.
Transfer the müesli into serving bowls and top each serving with the raspberries and sliced fresh banana, then serve.

—

TIP: Add some protein powder to make this a full breakfast meal. For busy mornings, prepare your müesli in a to-go cup to take with you.

200 g unsweetened müesli

200 mL whole milk yogurt or almond milk

1 tbsp. chia seeds

1 medium banana, peeled and mashed + more to serve

50 g raspberries

Ham and Avocado Sandwich with Cottage Cheese on Wheat Bread

Carefully scoop the flesh out of the avocado halves and slice them. Fan the slices out so they lay flat. Drizzle them with lime juice and sprinkle them with salt.

On each toasted bread slice, arrange the avocado slices and ham, then top with the cottage cheese and arugula. Drizzle them with olive oil, season with salt and pepper, then serve.

1 medium avocado, halved and pitted

Juice of 1 lime

2 slices bread, toasted

4 slices good-quality air-dried ham

50–75 g cottage cheese

1 generous handful fresh arugula, rinsed and dried, to serve

Olive oil, to serve

Salt and pepper, to taste

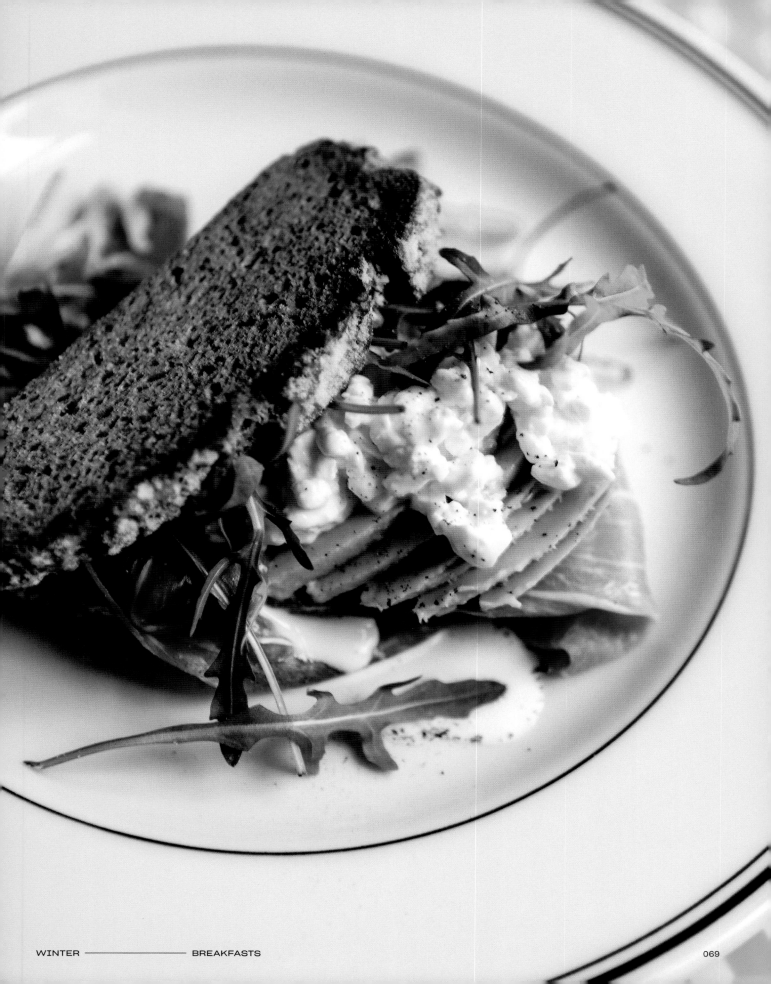

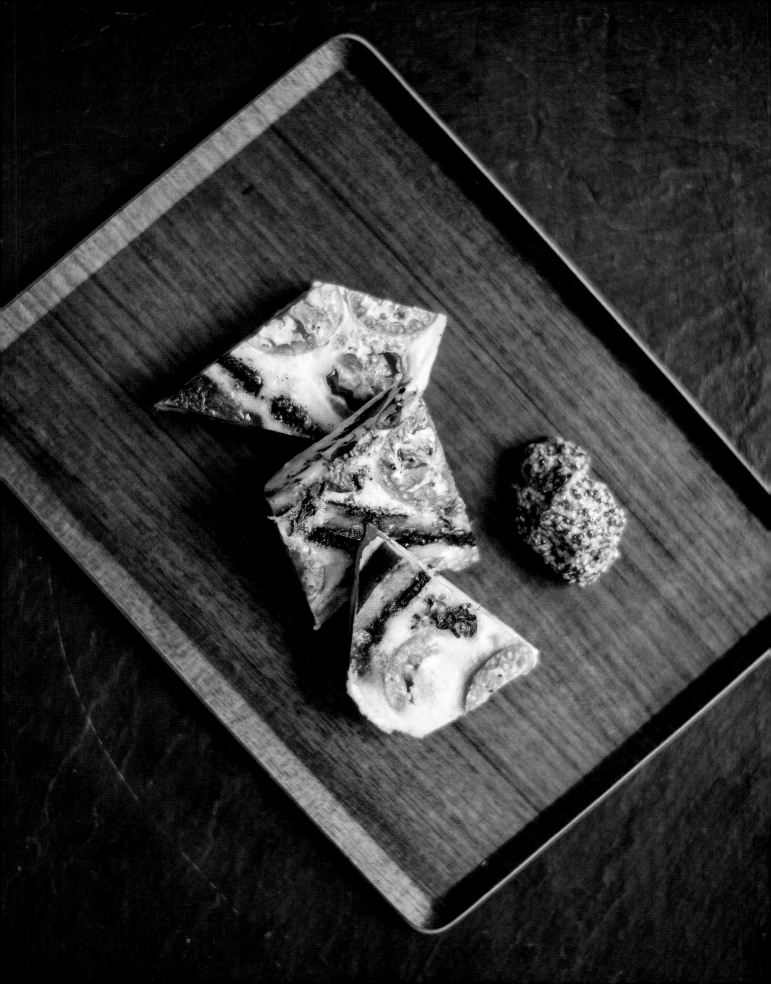

Frittata with Portobello Mushrooms, Tomatoes, and Basil

Preheat the oven to 170°C/335°F. Line a round cake pan with parchment paper and lightly grease both the pan and paper with oil. In a mixing bowl, whisk the eggs, then season with salt, pepper and nutmeg to taste. Set them aside. Rinse and slice the mushrooms and tomatoes into 1 cm-thick pieces. Heat up a pan with the olive oil and sprinkle it with salt. Fry the mushrooms until golden, then remove them from the heat.

———

Transfer the mushrooms, tomatoes and basil into the prepared pan. Pour the egg mixture over the vegetables and sprinkle with the Parmesan. Bake for 20–25 minutes until the egg mixture has set. Remove the pan from the oven and let it cool down for 10 minutes before slicing and serving with mustard on the side.

———

TIP: The frittata can be eaten cold as part of a portable lunch or a recovery meal with quinoa or rice on the side.

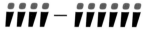

8 whole large eggs

Freshly grated nutmeg, to taste

Salt and pepper, to taste

2 portobello mushrooms,

100 g fresh tomatoes

1 tbsp. olive oil

1 bunch fresh basil

50 g freshly shredded Parmesan cheese

Dijon mustard, to serve

Pan-fried Redfish on Beets with Tangy Avocado Sauce

Rinse the beets and boil them in unsalted water for 30–40 minutes until tender. Let them cool down, put on single-use gloves, and squeeze their skins off. Slice them into bite-sized pieces and season with salt, pepper and balsamic vinegar. Set them aside.

—

Halve and pit the avocados. Scoop the flesh out and blend it with the lime juice, chili pepper and garlic until smooth. Add water if needed, then season with salt and pepper. Set the sauce aside.

—

Season the fish fillets with salt. Heat up a non-stick pan over medium heat with the olive oil. Place the fish skin-side down and fry for 1–2 minutes until they are about 80% cooked. Flip them over, remove them from the heat, and allow them to rest in the warm skillet for about 1 minute. If the fish is done, a cake tester should slide through the flesh easily.

—

Toss the coriander with the beets, then season with salt, pepper and balsamic vinegar to taste. Divide the mixture onto 2 plates and top each with a fish fillet. Pour 2 spoons of avocado sauce beside the fish and serve the rest on the side.

500 g beets

1 tbsp. balsamic vinegar + more to taste

1 medium avocado

Juice of 2 limes

1 medium green chili pepper

1 clove garlic, peeled

400 g redfish fillets, descaled and deboned

1 tbsp. olive oil

½ bunch of fresh coriander or cilantro

Salt and pepper, to taste

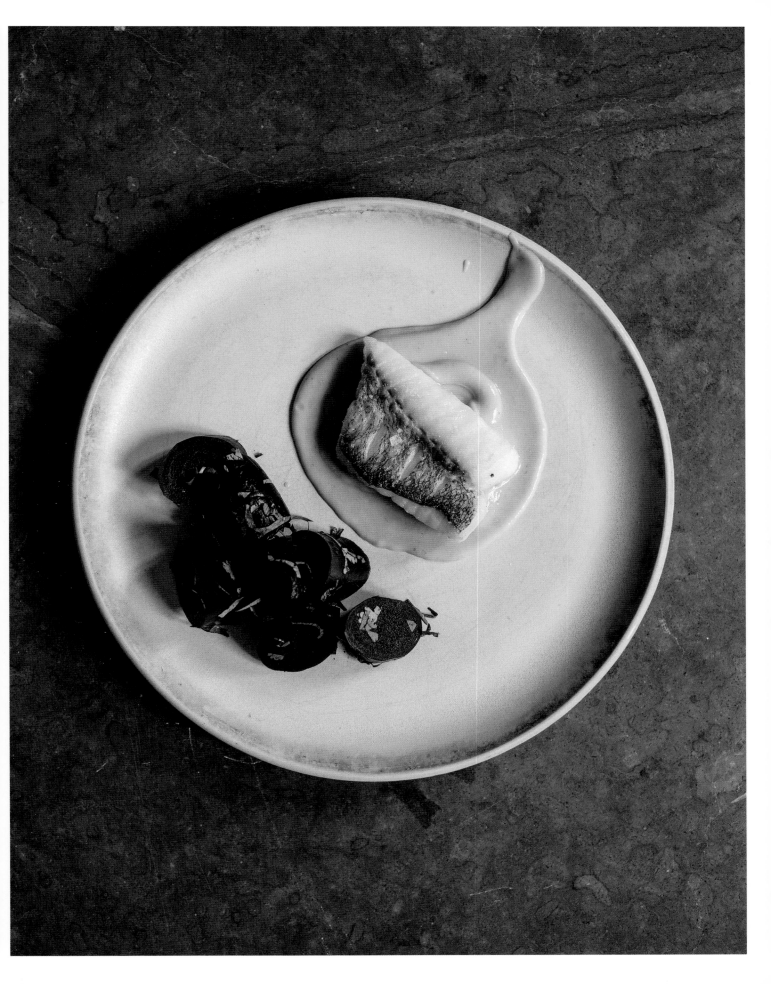

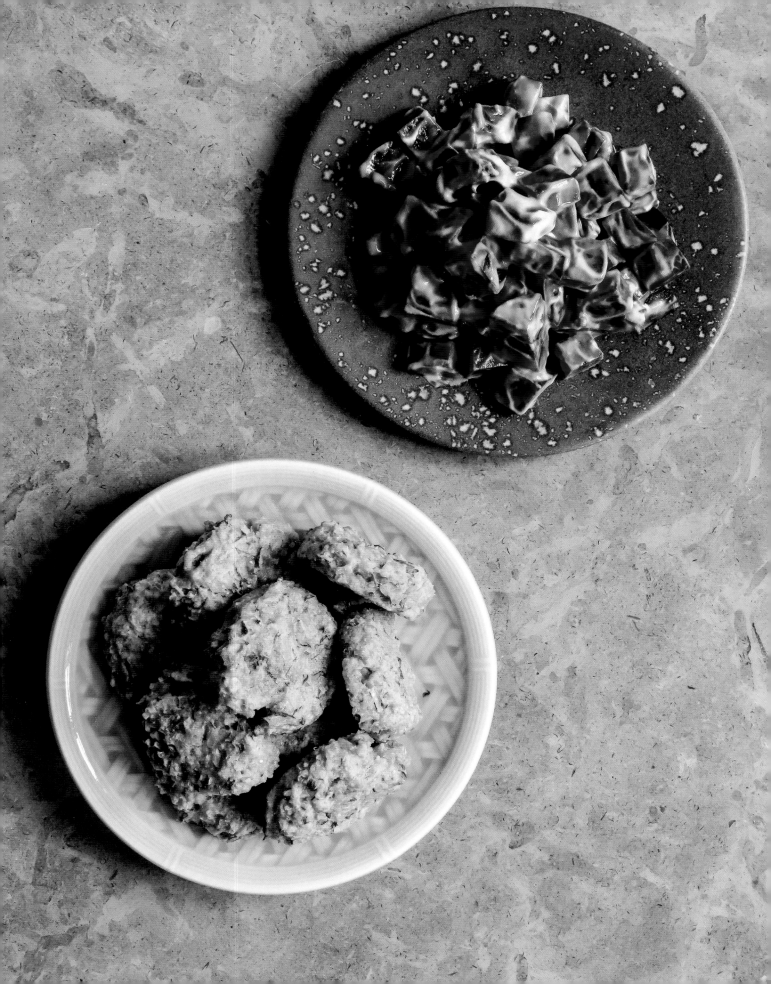

Quinoa Falafel in Salad Wraps with Beets in Spicy Yogurt

G D N

Preheat the oven to 240°C/475°F. Line a baking sheet with parchment paper. In a large pot over medium-high heat, bring the quinoa to a boil. Reduce the heat and cook uncovered for 10 minutes. Remove the pot from the heat, cover, and set it aside to steep for 5 minutes. Transfer the quinoa into a mixing bowl and let it cool down for at least 10 minutes.

———

Peel and mince the onion and garlic, then keep ½ of the garlic separate. Rinse and pick the parsley, then chop it coarsely. Peel the cooked beets and dice them. Add the onion, 1 clove of garlic, parsley, chickpea flour, cumin and egg to the quinoa, then stir until well combined. Season with lemon zest, juice, salt and pepper.

———

Shape the mixture into small falafel patties and place them onto the prepared sheet. Drizzle them with oil and bake for about 6 minutes. Flip them over and bake for another 6 minutes until golden. Remove them from the oven and set them aside. Combine the beets with the yogurt, ginger and remaining garlic. Season with salt, pepper and chili powder to taste. Serve the falafels with the beets on the side.

175 g cooked quinoa

350 mL lightly salted water

1 small onion

2 cloves garlic

1 handful fresh flat-leaf parsley

500 g cooked beets

45 g chickpea flour

1 g ground cumin

1 whole large egg

Zest and juice of 1 lemon

Salt and pepper, to taste

Olive oil, to bake

150 g plain Greek yogurt

10 g fresh ginger, minced

Chili powder, to taste

Braised Oxtails
with Ginger and Sichuan Pepper

G D N

Preheat the oven to 185°C/365°F. Peel the carrots, rinse and grate the ginger, halve the garlic heads horizontally, and slice the chili. Slice the cabbage thinly on a Japanese mandolin or using a sharp knife.

———

Cover the oxtails in oil and brown them thoroughly in the oven on a baking tray lined with parchment paper. Transfer them into a Dutch oven and turn the heat down to 160°C/320°F. Add the ginger, garlic, chili, star anise, maple/date syrup and Sichuan pepper, then sauté until the maple/date syrup is boiling and everything is glazed. Cut ⅓ of the carrots into bite-sized pieces and combine them with the oxtails. Add all the liquids, bring them to a boil over medium heat, place the Dutch oven in the oven covered, then cook for 3.5 hours until the meat is completely tender. Flip the oxtails in the braising liquid once every hour, so that they braise evenly.

———

Carefully remove the oxtails, garlic and carrots, then strain the liquid. Skim the surface and reduce the sauce to just about half. Add the oxtails, garlic and carrots back into the sauce, then season to taste with soy and rice vinegar. Heat up a pan with oil and roast the remaining carrots until golden and tender, then season with salt. Remove the carrots, wipe the pan clean with a paper towel and sauté the red cabbage until soft and tender. Season with rice vinegar and soy sauce. Serve the oxtails on rice with the roasted carrots and sautéed cabbage topped with coriander.

———

TIP: Leftover oxtail and cabbage make for great sandwich fillings the next day.

800 g carrots

50 g fresh ginger

2 whole heads of garlic

1 red chili

½ head red cabbage

1500 g oxtails

3 star anise

50 mL maple/date syrup

1–2 tsp. ground Sichuan pepper, to taste

200 mL sake or white wine

100 mL soy sauce or tamari

300 mL chicken broth or water

3 tbsp. rice vinegar

1 bunch fresh coriander or cilantro

Oil, to roast and cook

Steamed rice, to serve

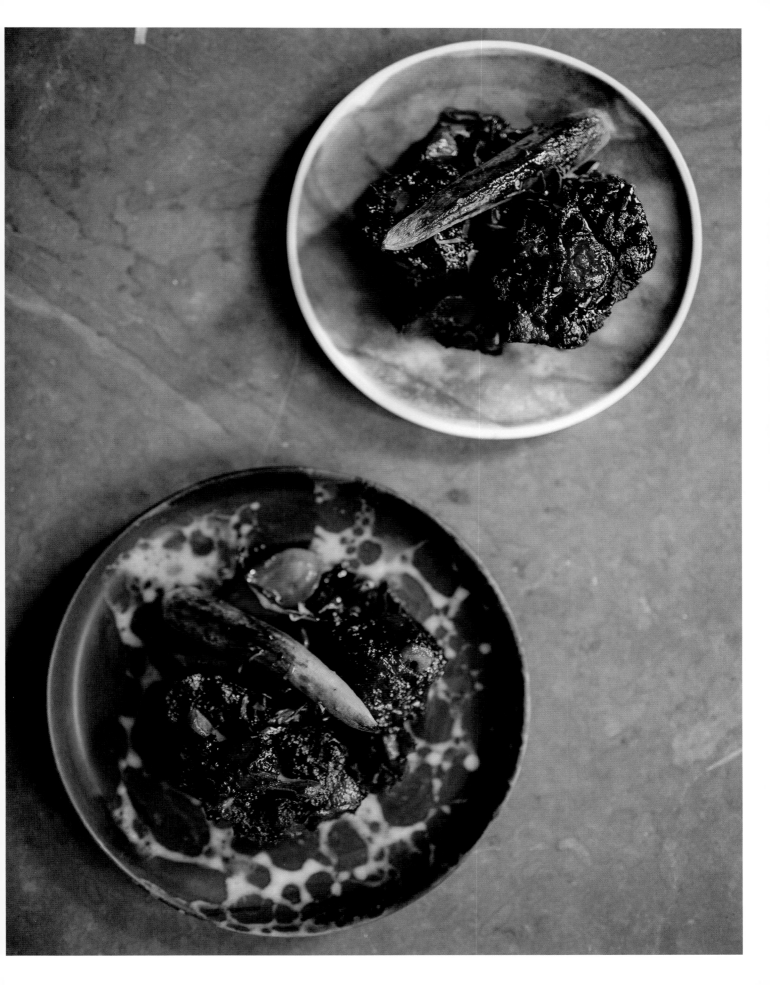

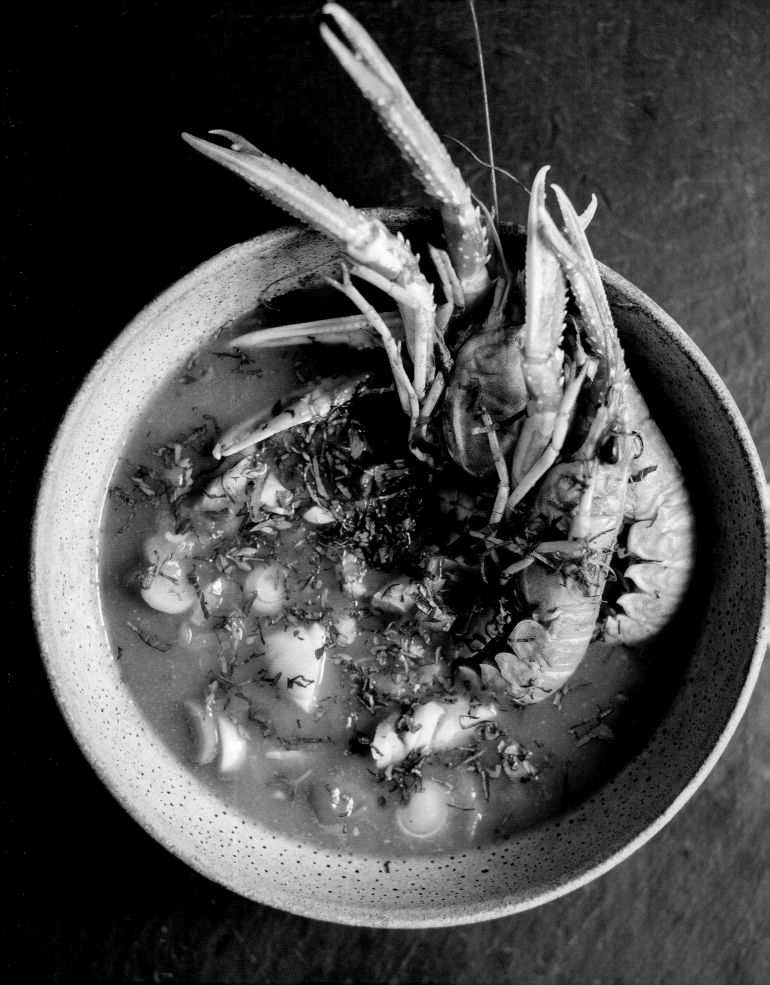

Fish Soup

Rinse all the vegetables. Slice the leeks and garlic, then dice the onion and fennel. Rinse and pick all the herbs separately, then slice the parsley thinly. Heat up a large pot with 1 tbsp. of olive oil. Add the leeks, garlic, onion, fennel and thyme, then sauté for about 2–3 minutes until the onion is tender and translucent. Add the tomato paste and cook for 1 minute. Add the wine and cook until the liquid reduces by half. Add the tomatoes and water, then season with salt and pepper. Bring it to a boil, then reduce the heat to medium-low amd simmer for about 20 minutes. Season with lemon zest, juice, nutmeg, salt and pepper to taste.

———

Remove any bones or scales from the fish and dice it into 3 cm x 3 cm cubes. Season them with salt and set them aside to cure for 20 minutes. Add the fish and langoustine tails to the soup, then gently bring it to a simmer. Remove the pot from the heat and set it aside to rest for 5 minutes. Transfer the soup into a large serving bowl and sprinkle with parsley. Serve hot with the bread on the side.

———

TIP: To carb up your meal, add dices of 1–2 baking potatoes towards the end of the cooking time and cook until tender.

2 medium leeks

3 cloves garlic

1 medium onion

1 medium fennel

½ bunch fresh thyme

½ bunch fresh flat-leaf parsley + more to serve

Olive oil, to cook

40 g tomato paste

250 mL white wine

2 cans crushed tomatoes

500 mL water

Salt and pepper, to taste

Zest and juice of 2 lemons

Freshly grated nutmeg, to taste

400 g fresh codfish, skinned

8–12 langoustine tails, rinsed

Bread, to serve

Spicy Ramen with Pickled Egg and Nori

Rinse all the vegetables. Peel and mince the ginger and garlic. Cut the bok choy into 6 or 8 wedges. Slice the spring onion and chili pepper. In a medium-sized stockpot over medium heat, heat up the olive oil. Add the ginger and garlic, then sauté for 1 minute. Add the broth and miso paste, then bring it to a boil. Poach the bok choy until vivid green and tender, then remove the pot from the heat. Season with lime zest, juice, tamari, chili paste and salt to taste.

In a frying pan over medium heat, caramelize the slices of chashu on both sides until golden and warm, then remove the pan from the heat. Divide the noodles into serving bowls, then pour the soup over them. Arrange the bok choy, chashu and eggs on top. Serve with spring onion, chili pepper, nori seaweed and pickled ginger.

25 g fresh ginger

4 cloves garlic

2 bok choy

1 bunch spring onions

1 red chili pepper

1 tbsp. olive oil

1 L chicken broth

50 g miso paste

Zest and juice of 2 limes

30 mL tamari

10–30 mL chili paste, to taste

Salt, to taste

8–12 slices chashu (see recipe on p.83)

Cooked noodles of your choice, to serve

4 ramen eggs, halved (see recipe on p.83)

4 sheets nori seaweed, cut into strips

50 g pickled ginger

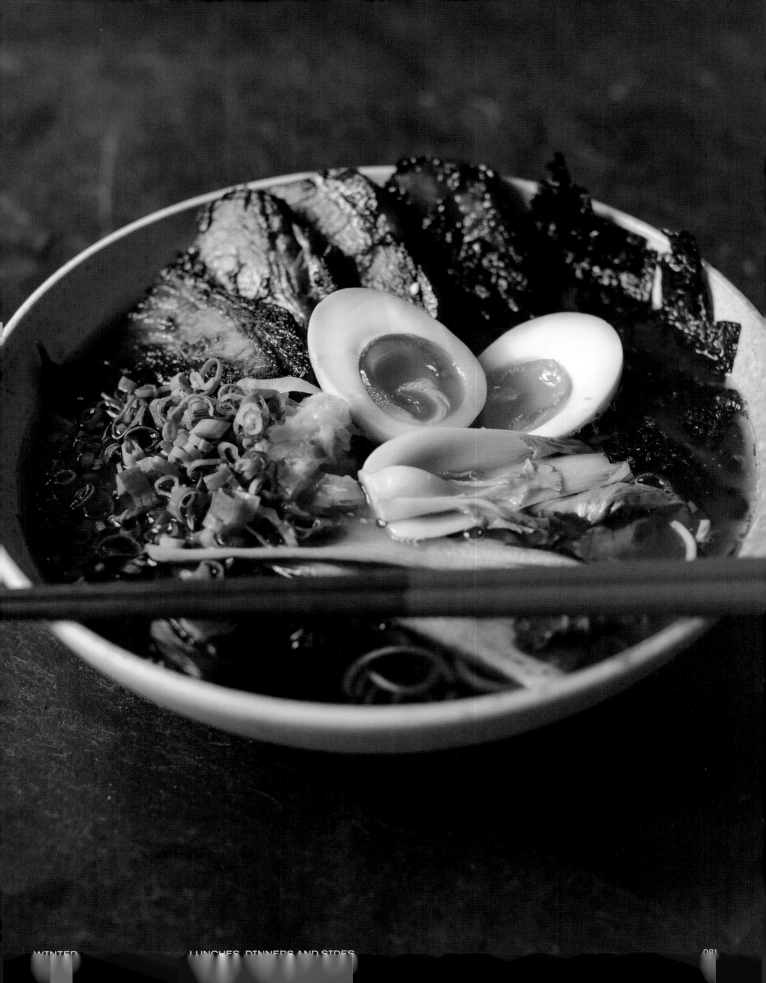

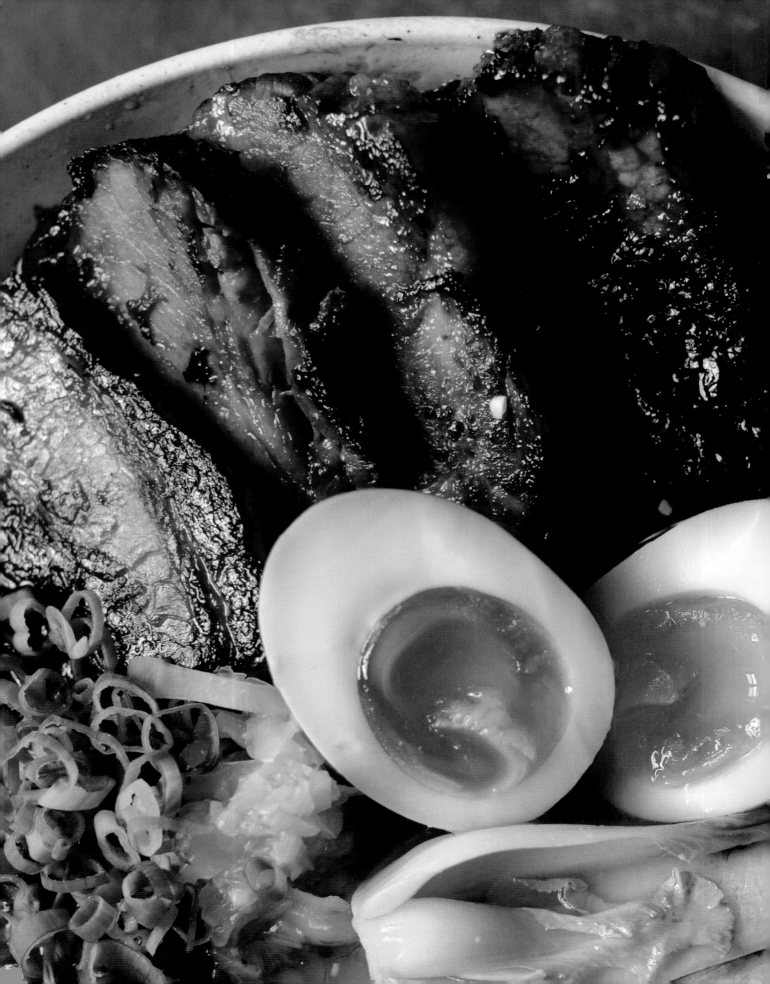

Pickled Eggs

Bring a large pot of water to a boil, submerge the eggs, and bring it to a boil again. Reduce the heat to medium-low and simmer until the desired consistency (see egg cooking times below). Remove the pot from the heat, and chill the eggs down in ice water. Once they have chilled, peel them.

In a small saucepan, combine the tamari, water and mirin, then bring them to a boil. Remove the pan from the heat and set it aside to cool down. Place the eggs into a plastic bag and pour the tamari liquid over them. Refrigerate the bag to marinate the eggs for at least 4 hours or overnight.

EGG COOKING TIMES
For a soft, runny yolk: 5 minutes
For a custard-like yolk: 6-8 minutes
Cooking times may vary depending on the eggs' size and freshness.

10 whole large eggs

200 mL tamari

200 mL water

100 mL mirin or
100 mL water with 2 tbsp. honey

Ramen Pork Chashu (Pork Belly)

Preheat the oven to 160°C/320°F. In a large frying pan over medium heat, caramelize the pork belly on all sides until golden and warm. Remove the pan from the heat.

In a medium ovenproof pot over medium-high heat, combine the water, soy sauce, sake, honey and sliced ginger, then bring them to a boil. Submerge the pork belly and the green parts of the scallions in the liquid, then return it to a boil. Place a piece of parchment paper over the pork belly and reduce the heat to medium-low. Place a couple of spoons on top of the parchment paper to keep the pork belly submerged and cook for about 15 minutes.

Remove the pot from the heat, and place it in the oven. Flip the pork belly occasionally while it cooks for about 1.5 hours until tender. Remove the pot from the oven and set it aside to cool slightly before slicing. Pan-sear the pork belly slices and serve with ramen or on steamed rice with vegetables.

500 g fresh pork belly

400 mL water

200 mL soy sauce

200 mL sake

45 g honey or sugar

50 g fresh ginger, thinly sliced

1 bunch fresh scallions

Coq au Vin Rouge with Brown Rice

Prepare the bouquet garni by placing all the ingredients into a single-use teabag. Preheat the oven to 175°C/345°F. In a Dutch oven, bring the wine, chicken broth and balsamic vinegar to a boil. Cook uncovered until its volume reduces by ⅓. Remove the Dutch oven from the heat.

———

Season the chicken pieces with salt and pepper. Heat up 2 tbsp. of olive oil in a frying pan. Caramelize the carrots, fennel, onions and garlic, then place them into the Dutch oven. Wipe the pan clean with a paper towel and heat it up over medium heat. Cook the chicken pieces skin-side down until golden brown. Transfer them into the Dutch oven skin-side up. Add the bouquet garni, fresh thyme sprigs and honey, then cover it with parchment paper and a lid. Cook for about 1 hour until the chicken is completely tender.

———

Discard the bouquet garni and thyme sprigs. Strain the Dutch oven liquid into a small saucepan over medium heat and reduce it down to about half. Season the sauce with salt, pepper and balsamic vinegar. Pour it over the chicken and vegetables. Garnish with lemon zest and thyme leaves, then serve with steamed brown rice.

For the Bouquet Garni:

5 sprigs fresh thyme, washed and picked

4 sprigs fresh rosemary, washed

1 tbsp. coriander seeds

2 bay leaves

5 cloves

1 star anise

For the Coq au Vin:

500 mL red wine

500 mL chicken broth

50 mL balsamic vinegar + more to taste

4 whole chicken legs,
divided into upper and lower thighs

Salt and pepper, to taste

30 mL olive oil

4 medium carrots, peeled

2 medium bulbs fennel, cut into wedges

2 medium onions,
peeled and cut into wedges

1 whole bulb garlic, halved horizontally

30 mL honey

5–6 sprigs fresh thyme or lemon thyme
+ more to serve

Zest of 2 lemons

Steamed brown rice, to serve

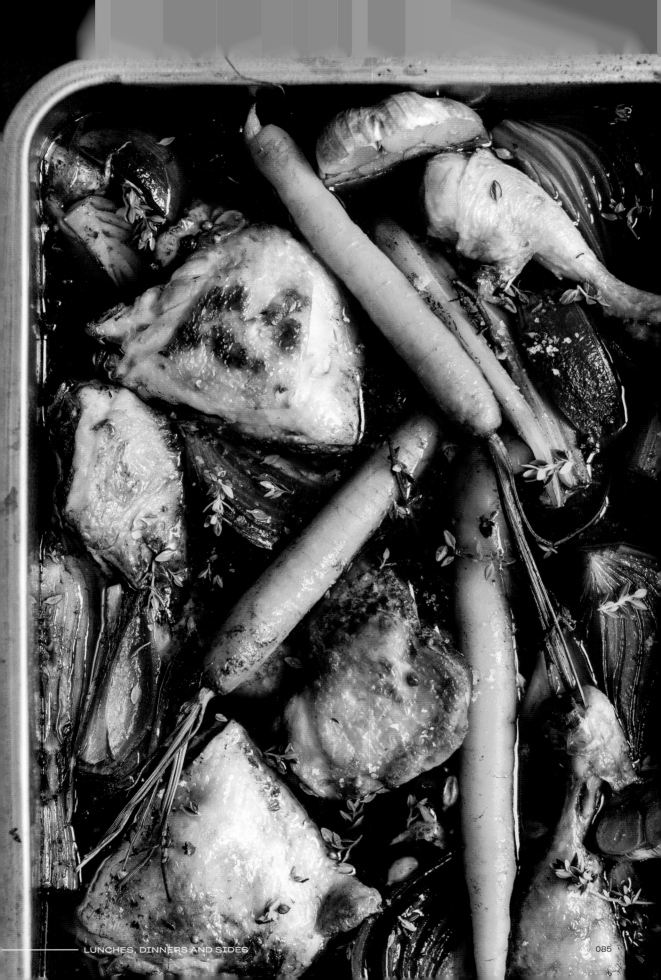

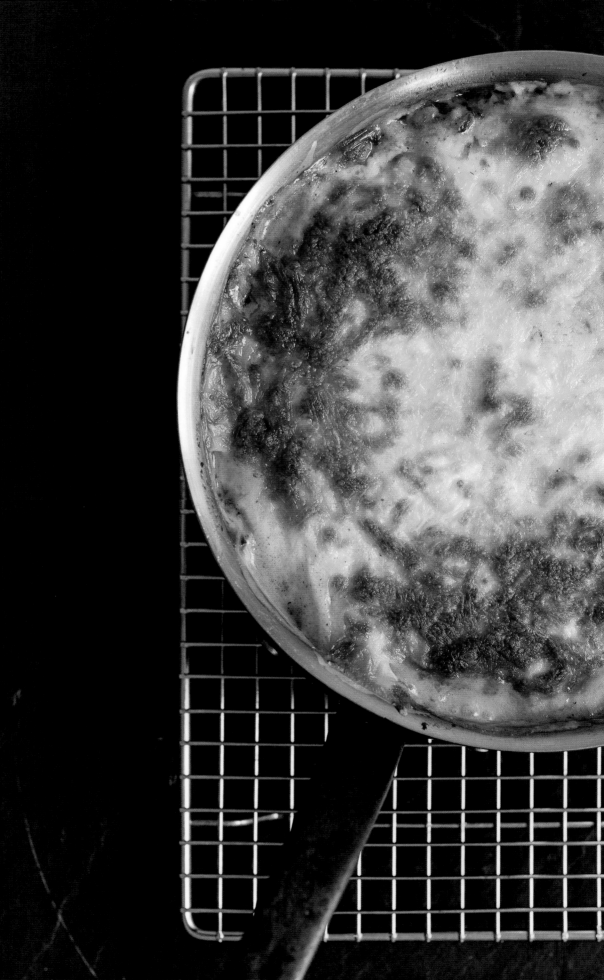

Moussaka

Heat up 2 tbsp. of olive oil in a large pot and brown the meat. Add the onions and garlic, then sauté until the onions are soft. Add the tomatoes, carrots, balsamic vinegar, tomato paste, oregano and cinnamon, then season with salt and pepper. Bring the meat sauce to a boil, then reduce the heat to low and let it simmer covered. Stir occasionally for 20 minutes, remove the pot from the heat and season again with salt and pepper if necessary.

Heat up the milk in a casserole until it is warm, not boiling. In a small mixing bowl, whisk the corn starch and water together, then whisk the mixture into the warm milk as you bring it to a boil over medium heat. Keep whisking for 3 minutes until the milk sauce is nice and thick. Remove the casserole from the heat, add the Parmesan, then season with salt, pepper and nutmeg to taste.

Preheat the oven to 175°C/345°F. In an ovenproof baking dish, layer the meat sauce, milk sauce, and sliced vegetables - starting and ending with the milk sauce. Season each layer of vegetable with salt and pepper. Top with mozzarella and bake for 1 hour and 15 minutes until golden brown and the potatoes are tender. Serve it straight from the oven.

Olive oil, to cook

400 g ground veal, beef, or lamb

2 medium onions, peeled and diced

4 cloves garlic, minced

2 cans (800 g) crushed tomatoes

2 large carrots, shredded

45 mL balsamic vinegar

40 g tomato paste

1 tsp. dried oregano

1 pinch ground cinnamon

Salt and pepper, to taste

1 L whole milk

50 mL water

20 g cornstarch

100 g freshly shredded Parmesan cheese

Freshly grated nutmeg, to taste

1 medium eggplant (aubergine), thinly sliced on a mandolin

2 medium baking potatoes, thinly sliced on a mandolin

1 medium squash, thinly sliced on a mandolin

50 g shredded mozzarella

Grilled Eggplant, Tomatoes, and Mozzarella

Preheat the oven to 170°C/340°F. Toast the pine nuts for about 15 minutes until golden. Heat up a large sauté pan with 2 tbsp. of olive oil. Add the onions, garlic and thyme, then sauté for 2 minutes until the onions are soft. Add the tomatoes, balsamic vinegar, tomato paste, bay leaves and star anise, then bring them to a boil. Reduce the heat to medium-low and simmer for 10 minutes until the tomato sauce has thickened. Discard the star anise and bay leaves, then season with salt, pepper and balsamic vinegar to taste. Remove the pan from the heat.

Cut the tops off each eggplant, slice them into 1 cm-thick pieces and sprinkle them lightly with salt. Warm a large pan or grill pan over high heat and fry them in a little bit of olive oil until dark brown. Keep the eggplant warm on a plate under tin foil. Wipe the pan clean with a paper towel and heat it up with ½ tbsp. of olive oil. Sprinkle it with salt, then cook the spinach and basil quickly. Keep the spinach warm on a plate under tin foil as well. Slice the mozzarella into 1 cm-thick pieces and heat up the pan again at medium-high heat. Caramelize the mozzarella for about 30-45 seconds. To serve, stack the eggplant, tomato sauce, spinach, and mozzarella into towers, then sprinkle them with the pine seeds.

50 g pine nuts

Olive oil, to cook

2 medium onions, peeled and minced

3 cloves garlic, peeled and minced

½ bunch fresh thyme, finely chopped

800 g fresh tomatoes, diced or 2 cans (400 g)

45 mL balsamic vinegar + more to taste

40 g tomato paste

2 bay leaves

1 star anise

4 medium eggplants

200 g fresh spinach, washed

1 bunch fresh basil, washed

250 g fresh mozzarella

Salt and pepper, to taste

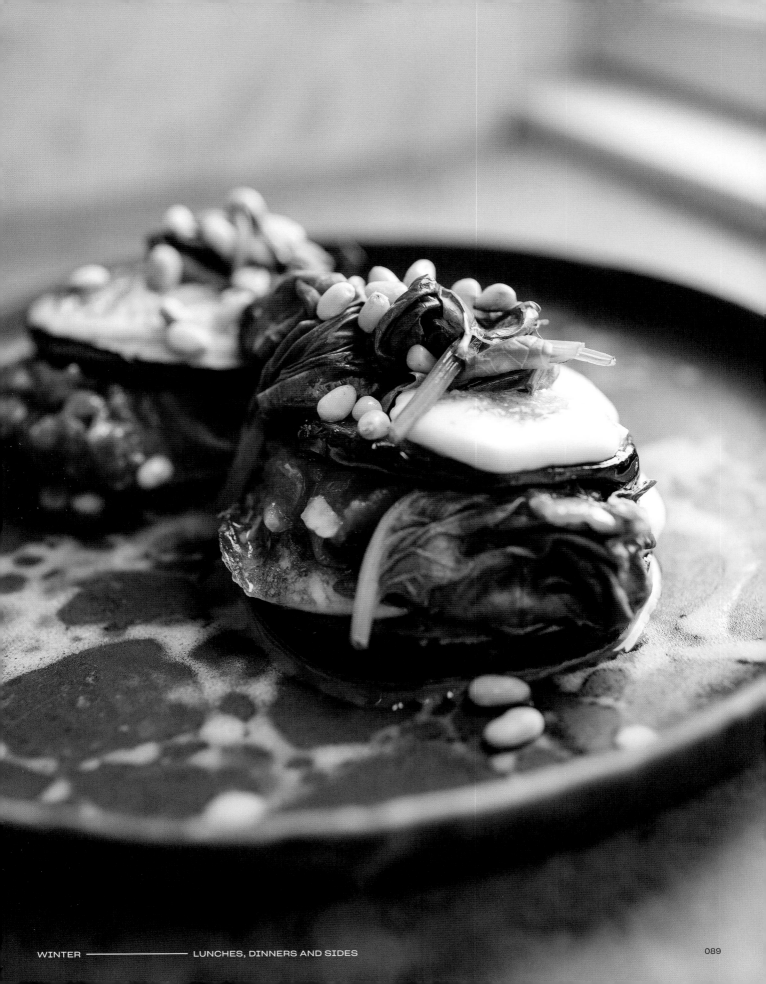

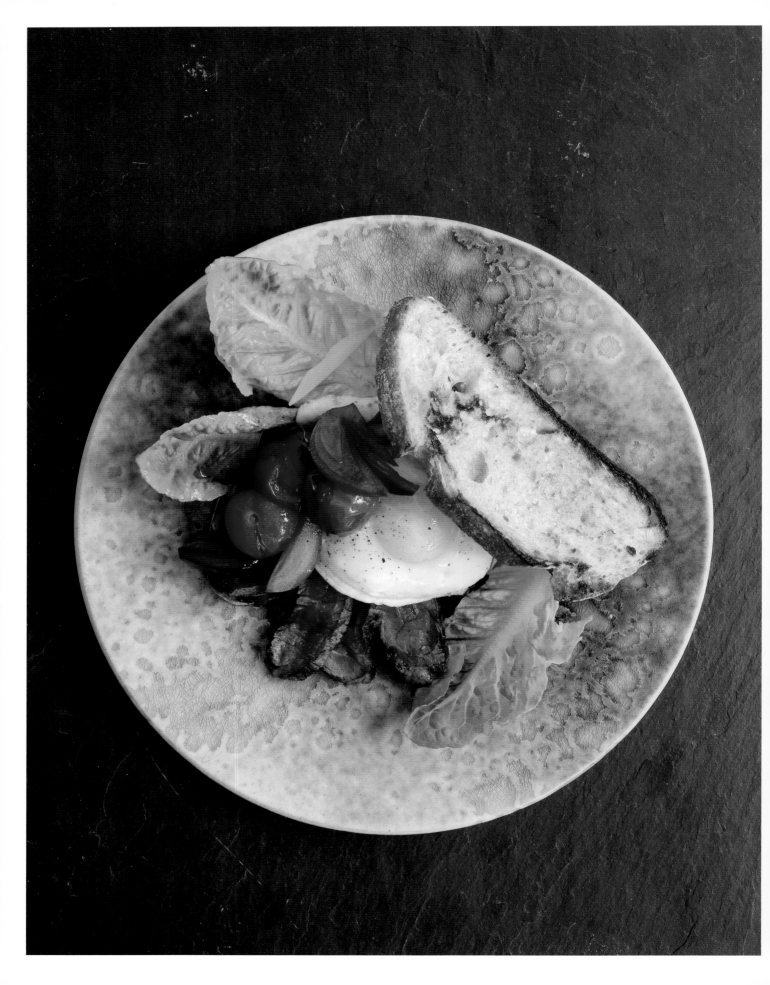

Veal Steak and Egg Sandwiches with Pickled Tomato and Onion

Rinse and pierce a hole in each tomato with a small knife. Peel the onions and slice them into wedges. Transfer them onto a casserole and add the 50 mL of olive oil, balsamic vinegar, ½ tsp. of salt, star anise and rosemary. Slowly bring it all to a boil, remove the pot from the heat and let it sit for at least 15 minutes or refrigerate in an airtight container for 4–5 days.

———

Season the steaks with salt and pepper. In a large frying pan over medium-high heat, heat up 1 tbsp. of olive oil, and fry them for 2–3 minutes on each side. Place them on a cutting board and let them rest for 5 minutes before slicing. Season the slices with salt and pepper. Wipe the pan clean with a paper towel and heat it up with 1 tbsp. of olive oil. Fry 2 eggs over medium heat until the egg white has set.

———

Toast the bread slices. Spread the mustard thinly on each toasted slice, then top with lettuce leaves and steak slices. Serve with the pickled tomato and onion, a fried egg per slice and Parmesan.

200 g cherry tomatoes

1 medium red onion

50 mL + 2 tbsp. olive oil

50 mL. balsamic vinegar

1 star anise

2 sprigs fresh rosemary

2 veal steaks (150 g each)

2 whole eggs

4 slices bread

2 tbsp. Dijon mustard

1 little gem lettuce,
leaves separated and rinsed

50 g freshly shaved Parmesan cheese

Salt and pepper, to taste

Chicken Tsukune
with Yuke and Shaved Cabbage Salad

GDN

ii – iiii

Preheat the oven to 200°C/390°F. Line a baking tray with parchment paper. Soak 12 wooden skewers in water to prevent them from burning in the oven.

In a mixing bowl, mix the chicken, onion, shiso, ginger and garlic by hand. Add the tamari and season with salt, then gently mix until well combined. Fry a small portion of raw tsukune to taste if the seasoning needs tweaking, and adjust accordingly. Shape into 10–12 oblong meatballs. Pierce the meatballs with the skewers and brush them with oil. Place them on the prepared tray and bake for about 8–10 minutes until the meat is firm and fully cooked through. Remove the tray from the oven.

Discard any damaged or dirty outer leaves from the cabbages. Shave them thinly on a Japanese mandolin or using a sharp knife. In a large bowl, massage the shaved cabbage with the rice wine vinegar and pinch of salt. Mix in the mint.

In small serving dishes, place the yolks and tamari. Whisk them together into a yuke sauce just before eating. Serve the skewers with the shaved cabbage and yuke sauce on the side.

400 g ground chicken

1 small red onion, peeled and minced

10 g finely sliced fresh shiso leaf or mint

20 g fresh ginger, peeled and minced

2 cloves garlic, peeled and minced

20 mL tamari + 100 mL tamari to serve, divided

Salt, to taste

Olive oil, to bake

½ medium summer cabbage

½ medium red cabbage

1 tbsp. rice wine vinegar

1 pinch salt

1 bunch fresh mint, rinsed and thinly sliced

2 egg yolks, to serve

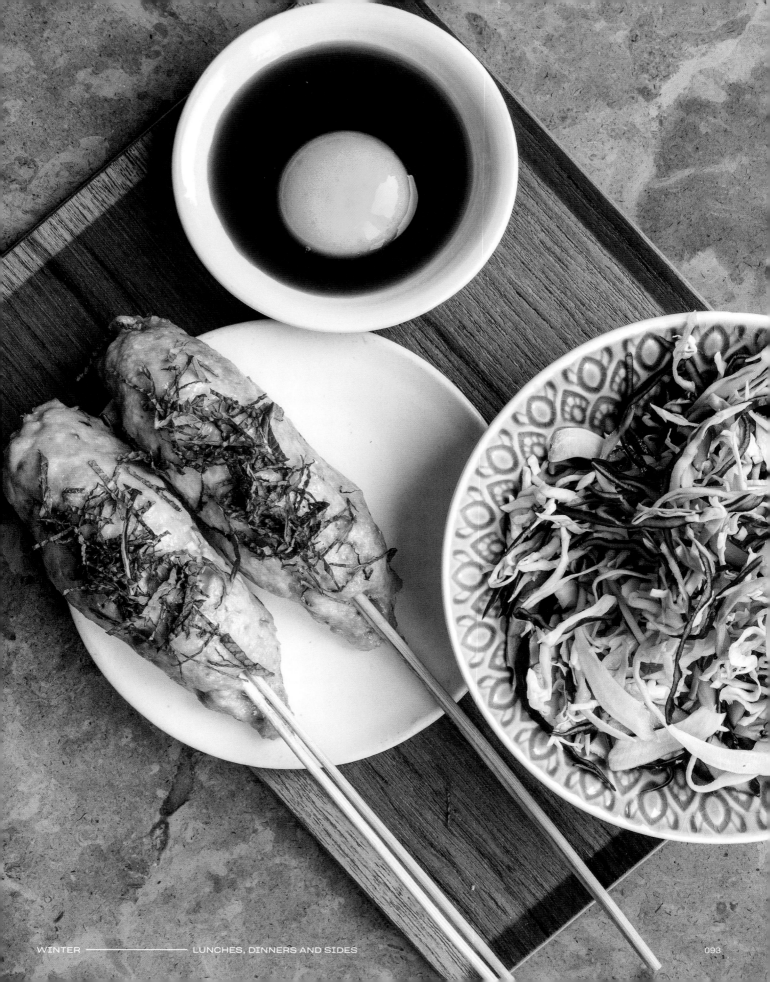

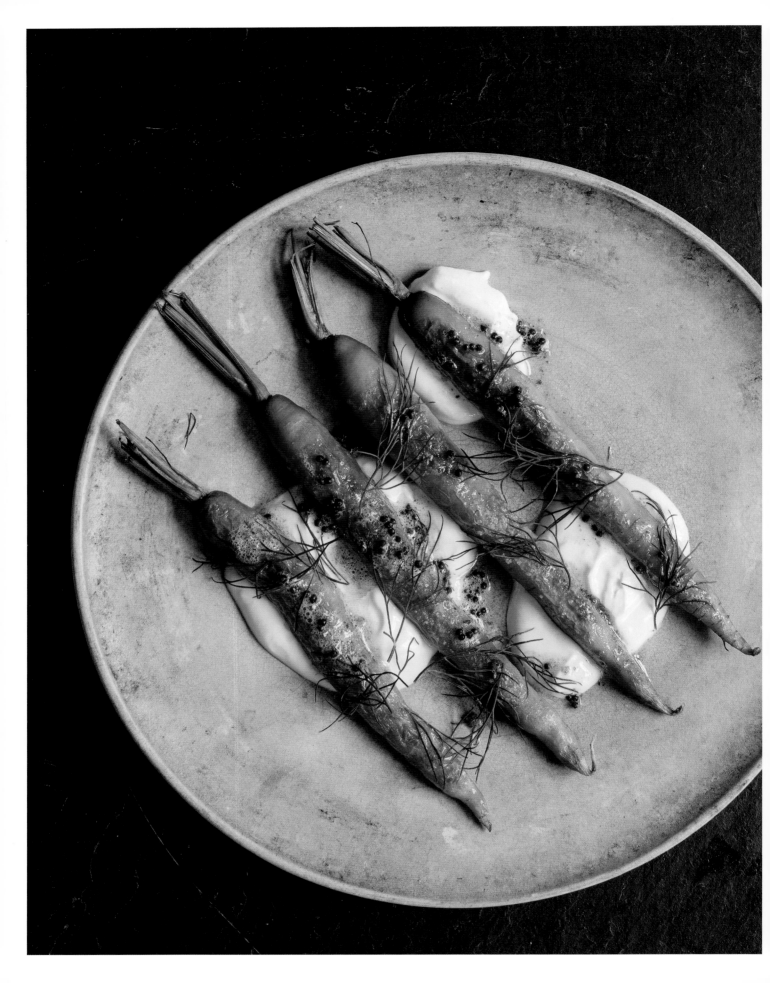

Whole Roasted Carrots
with Brown-butter Vinaigrette, Dill, and Yogurt

 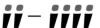

In a small casserole over medium-low heat, melt the butter. Cook until the whey (milk solids) caramelizes, and the butter smells nutty and looks golden brown. Whisk in the mustard seeds, 25 mL of olive oil and apple cider vinegar, then let them simmer over low heat for 5 minutes.

———

Heat up a frying pan with the remaining olive oil. Roast the carrots over medium-high heat until golden brown and tender, then season with salt and pepper to taste. Season the yogurt with salt to taste, then arrange 3 spoons of it on a serving platter and place the carrots on top. Drizzle the brown-butter vinaigrette over the carrots and top them with the picked dill, then serve.

25 g butter

2 tbsp. mustard seeds

25 mL olive oil + 1 tbsp. olive oil, divided

25 mL apple cider vinegar + more to taste

500 g carrots,
scrubbed and split lengthwise

100 mL whole milk yogurt

1 bunch fresh dill, rinsed and picked

Salt and pepper, to taste

Oven-roasted Root Vegetables

Preheat the oven to 185°C/365°F. Line a baking sheet with parchment paper. Peel the carrots, beets and celery root, then cut them into bite-sized pieces. Rinse and pick the thyme. Toss the root vegetables with the olive oil, then season with salt and pepper. Transfer them onto the prepared sheet and bake for about 25–30 minutes until golden and tender. Top with lemon zest and picked thyme leaves. Serve on the side with a meat or fish dish.

—

TIP: Cook extra root vegetables for future use in a frittata (see recipe on p.99).

500 g carrots

500 g beets

500 g celery root

½ bunch fresh thyme

2 tbsp. olive oil

Salt and pepper, to taste

Zest and juice of 1 lemon

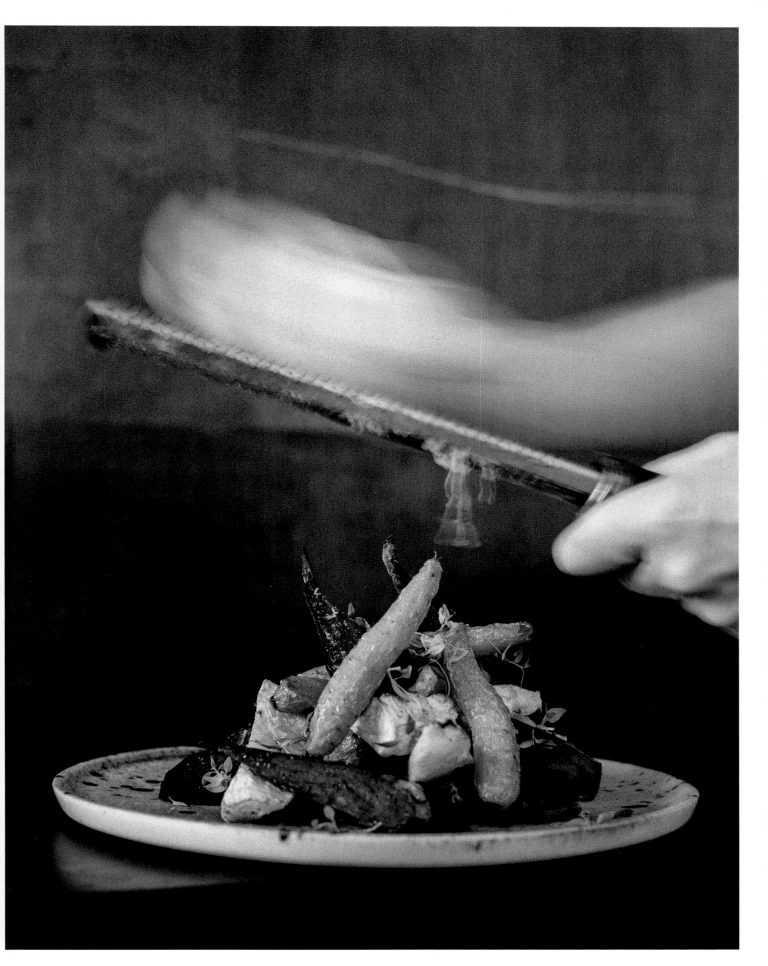

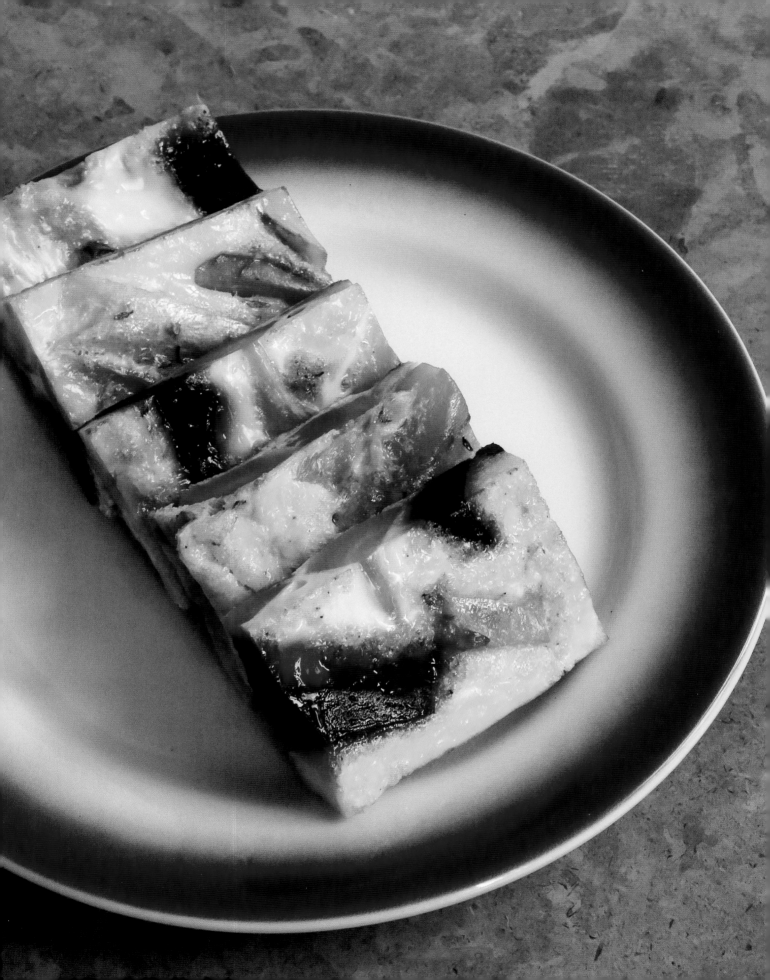

Oven-roasted Root Vegetable Frittata

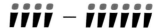

Preheat the oven to 170°C/340°F. Place the roasted root vegetables in a deep pie dish lined with greased parchment paper. Peel and slice the onions thinly. Heat up a frying pan with the olive oil and sauté the onions for 2–3 minutes until they are soft and sweet. Season with salt and pepper, then mix in the root vegetables.

In a large mixing bowl, whisk the eggs. Add the thyme, then season with salt, pepper and nutmeg to taste. Whisk until well combined. Pour the egg mixture over the root vegetables and bake for about 20 minutes until the egg has completely set. Remove the dish from the oven and let it cool down completely. Serve the frittata warm or cold with the mustard and green salad.

600 g mixed roasted root vegetables, cut into bite-sized pieces (see page 096)

2 onions

1 tbsp. olive oil

8 whole large eggs

½ bunch fresh thyme or rosemary

Salt and pepper, to taste

Freshly grated nutmeg, to taste

Dijon mustard, to serve

Green salad, to serve

Natasha's Beet Soup

GNV

Peel the carrots, onion, and garlic. Slice the onion and garlic, then julienne the carrots (into matchstick-sized strips). Core and slice the pepper and chili pepper. Peel and dice the beets, apples and potatoes. Dice the tomatoes. Slice the cabbage. Pick and chop the parsley and dill.

Heat up the oil in a large soup pot, then sauté the carrots, onion, garlic, pepper, and chili pepper for about 5 minutes until the onion is soft and tender. Add the beets, tomatoes, ½ of the broth and the tomato paste, then bring them to a boil. Reduce the heat to medium-low and simmer for about 20 minutes. Add the potatoes and cook for another 10-15 minutes over low heat until the potatoes are tender. Add the remaining broth, cabbage and apples, then simmer for 5-7 minutes. Season with apple cider vinegar, salt and pepper, then remove the pot from the heat. Serve in soup bowls, topped with sour cream, parsley, dill and lemon zest.

TIP: Make the soup 1 day ahead and refrigerate overnight to allow the flavors to meld.

200 g carrots

1 large onion

3 cloves garlic

1 medium sweet pepper

1 medium chili pepper

500 g beets

3 medium apples

2 baking potatoes

450 g ripe tomatoes

1 medium head pointed cabbage

1 bunch fresh flat-leaf parsley

1 bunch fresh dill, rinsed

1 L beef broth, divided

40 g tomato paste

100 mL sour cream or plain Greek yogurt

Salt and pepper, to taste

Apple cider vinegar, to taste

Zest of 2 lemons

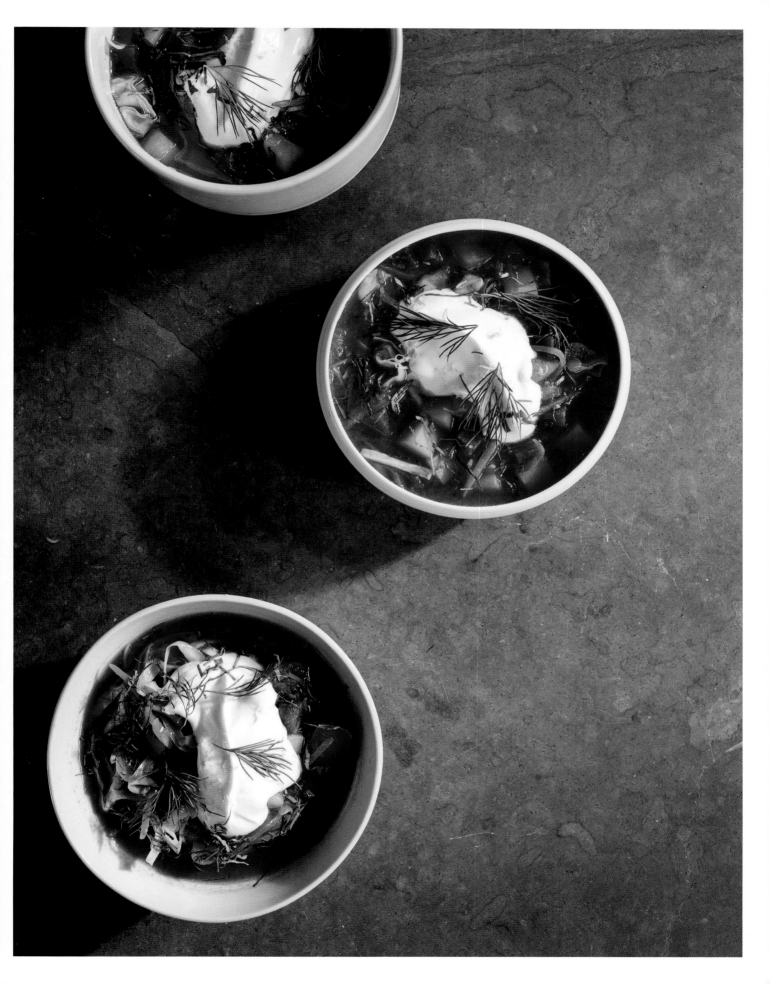

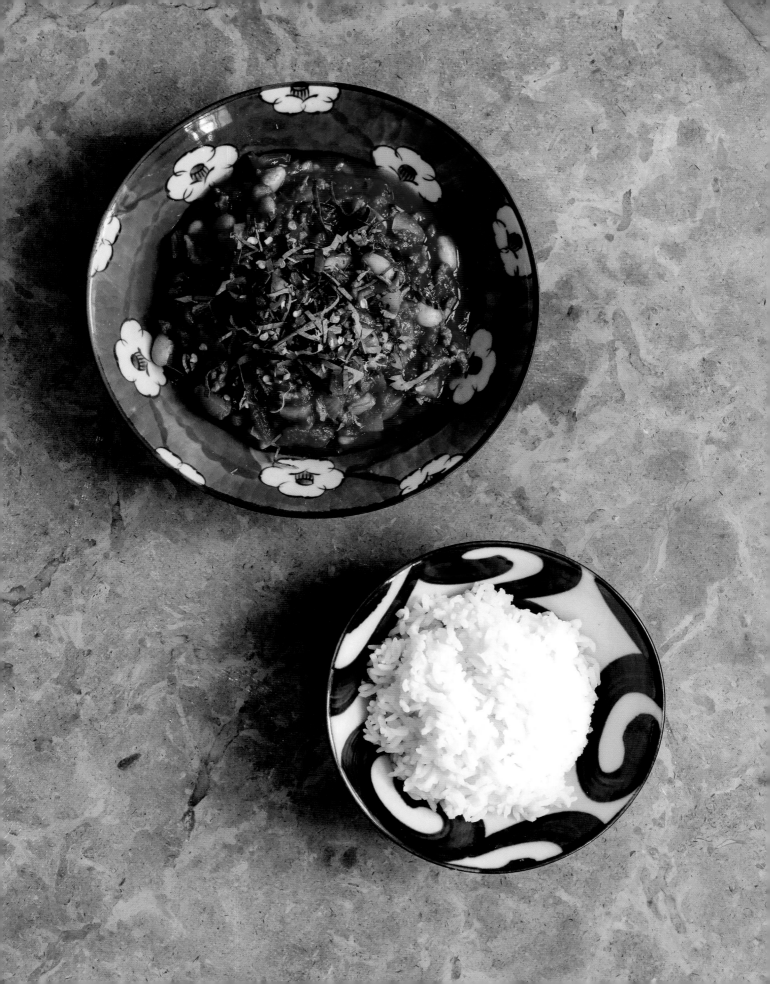

Chili con Carne

Rinse and peel all the vegetables. Dice the onions and fennel, then shred the carrots. Slice the garlic and celery thinly. Dice the tomatoes (if not canned) and slice the chili pepper.

———

Heat up a large soup pot with the olive oil, sprinkle it with salt and brown the ground beef well. Add the onions, fennel, carrots and garlic, then sauté for 5-7 minutes until the onions are soft and tender. Add the tomatoes, beans, water, balsamic vinegar, tomato paste, cumin, cocoa powder, oregano and chili flakes. Season with salt and pepper to taste, then bring them to a boil. Reduce the heat to medium-low and cook for 45 minutes, stirring occasionally until the chili is thick. Season with balsamic vinegar, salt and pepper to taste. Serve in bowls with steamed white rice, topped with parsley, coriander, lemon zest and chili pepper slices.

———

TIP: For a vegetarian variation (chili sin carne), follow this same process but substitute the ground beef for finely diced celery root.

3 medium onions

1 medium fennel bulb

2 medium carrots

5 cloves garlic

1 celery stalk

800 g whole tomatoes or 2 cans (400 g)

1 fresh chili pepper

2 tbsp. olive oil

400 g ground beef

400 g cooked white beans

100 mL water

30 mL balsamic vinegar + more to taste

25 g tomato paste

1 tsp. ground cumin

1 tbsp. unsweetened cocoa powder

1 tbsp. dried oregano

Chili flakes, to taste

1 bunch fresh flat-leaf parsley

½ bunch fresh coriander or cilantro

Zest of 1 lemon

Salt and pepper, to taste

Steamed white rice, to serve

Beet and Kale Salad
with Pistachios and Orange Dressing

G D N V

Peel and grate the beets. Wash and cut the kale into bite-sized pieces. Chop the pistachios. Peel and mince the garlic.

In a small mixing bowl, combine the garlic, orange zest and juice, white wine vinegar, honey and cinnamon. Season with salt and pepper to taste, then gradually drizzle in the olive oil.
Whisk constantly until the dressing is emulsified and thick. Season with salt, pepper and white wine vinegar if needed. Toss the beets and kale in ½ of the dressing. Plate the salad and sprinkle it with the pistachios. Serve the remaining dressing on the side.

600 g beets

200 g kale

20 g pistachios

1 clove garlic

Zest and juice of 2 oranges

3 tbsp. white wine vinegar + more to taste

1 tbsp. honey

1 pinch ground cinnamon

100 mL olive oil

Salt and pepper, to taste

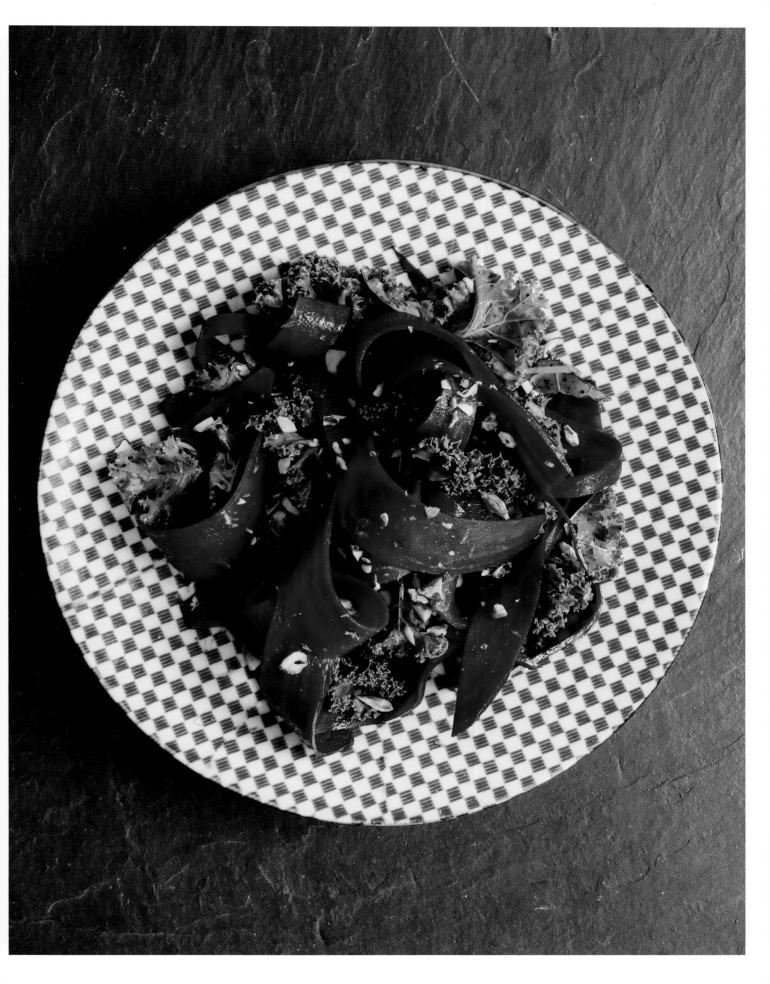

ERW
SPRING

Spring Breakfasts

Spring Lunches, Dinners and Sides

Sprouting

SPRING: TRAINING SEASON

In spring, daylight appears a little bit earlier, and cold mornings blend into warmer afternoons. This is the time to kick-start planned training and find your second gear, as early season races and events beckon around the corner. Unfortunately, this is also the time for you to head back outside and greet your allergies!

This section was carefully put together to support your increasing levels of physical activity and training output, as well as to reduce inflammation and seasonal allergies. You will find dishes that feature fresh young spring produce, whole grains, lean protein, and healthy fats like olive oil, nuts, and avocados to help you get fitter and leaner, stay healthy, and recover well.

Eat Race Win! Keywords for Spring

- New greens, root vegetables, seasonal fruits (no dried fruits other than dates)

- New potatoes, buckwheat, purple and red rice, rice noodles, mung bean noodles, rice papers, sweet potatoes

- Moderate amounts of animal fats (butter is good)

- Moderate amounts of coconut oil

- Olive and rice bran oils

- Lighter sources of protein, including poultry, fish, and lean proteins

- Nuts and seeds

- Sprouted foods, including chickpeas, mung beans, and almonds

- Other starches mixed with vegetables

MICHAEL
VALGREN
ANDERSEN

Born — 7 Feburary 1992
Professional since — 2014
Origin — Denmark
Lives in — Monte Carlo

Michael is the leader of a new breed of Vikings who are set to take cycling by storm. At just 26, his palmarès mark him out for future glory: he's a two-time winner of the Tour of Denmark and the junior Liège-Bastogne-Liège, as well as a national road race champion who enjoyed a breakthrough season in 2018 with victories in the Omloop Het Nieuwsblad and Amstel Gold Race (his "greatest victory" to-date).

I first met him when we were both with the Tinkoff-Saxo team, where he wore the Danish national champions jersey and some best young rider jerseys before moving on to the Astana team. I know he used to enjoy my cooking, so I wanted to find out how one of today's best young cyclists prepares for the season using diet and nutrition.

"Nutrition questions are always hard to answer because you change your diet many times during a season due to new rumors and science," Michael tells me. "That said, I always try to get a good solid breakfast like oats, and I often make porridge!" When training, he either stops en route and eats a sandwich, or makes a proper lunch at home beforehand. And what does he rustle up for himself? "Usually, a salad with tuna, eggs, and some pasta or bread with it. For dinner, I love to make steamed spinach with some kind of fish."

Michael laments that he's one of those people who only has to look at a cake or some ice cream to gain weight. "That's why eating healthily is the way forward for me, and I'm always really careful - or I try, at least!" He mentions his tendency to pile on the pounds over the winter, "but luckily, I'm gaining less weight as I gain more experience. There were some years when I'd gain between 7-9 kilos!"

What really works, he says, is to consume plenty of carbs for breakfast and after rides to perform well the next day. He has also changed his eating habits when he is out for a training ride. "This year, I started eating a lot more during my rides, which made them a lot better. I didn't have to binge eat when I got home. Before this, I didn't always eat or drink during a ride, so I felt like I could treat myself afterwards - but that just made my training and recovery really bad, and I couldn't perform well." So does eating a certain diet have any impact on his performance? "I don't feel such a big difference, but of course, if I were to eat junk food for a month, I'd probably feel like sh*t!"

Michael tells me he trains and races on a combination of real food such as homemade rice bars and jam or Philadelphia and ham sandwiches for the first 3-4 hours, before turning to engineered nutrition in the form of gels. "When the heat is on, I just eat gels because they're easy to take. During races, I don't eat anything new much: it's pasta, pasta, pasta. At home however, I eat a lot healthier and less, unlike how I used to eat when I was 'young'!"

"...eating healthily is the way forward for me, and I'm always really careful — or I try, at least!"

Michael acknowledges that eating healthy is a key component for performance, but he has a secret. "Actually, before an important race, I often eat candy," he laughs. "It's something that just has been working for me, so I save it for the important races. Back in 2013, when I was with my old continental team, we went out and bought a lot of candy on the day before the Danish championship - and ended up kicking all the pros' *sses! Since then, I've bought what we call 'winner candy' before important races." However, his favorite race food is rice bars from his own recipes: "We've just made some new ones with blueberry and chocolate chips in them. Really amazing! During races, I get 'acid burps' easily if I eat too much, so the rice bars are good for my stomach." So what works best for him on an important race day, besides candy and rice bars? "Oatmeal, müesli with coconut milk, an omelet with ham and cheese, and a ton of coffee - then I'm ready!" he grins. Post-racing, Michael has some carbs, a shower, and a protein shake. "I'd have pasta or rice with chicken for dinner, and a salad if the chef has prepared a nice one."

I wonder aloud if the taste and appearance of food is important to him on a long-stage race, where riders tend to lose their appetites. "For sure, taste is important, but I think we eat a lot more with our eyes," Michael replies. "If a dish is well made and looks great, we get total satisfaction!" What are his favorite foods in and out of season? "I love salmon and a proper risotto. Pasta. A good homemade burger. I'm a dressing guy, so whenever we make burgers, I have at least 5 different kinds of dips and sauces." He tells me that his best food experiences in the professional peloton were my rest day meals, "especially when you made burgers!" And the worst food ever? "When I was a junior riding in the Peace Race in Czech Republic, I had some really sh*tty pasta with cacao powder on top. It was so weird and strange!"

We talk about whether meal timings matter, and if he plans anything differently depending on the season. He shares that when he goes out for dinner with his fiancé, he often eats the contents of the bread basket before any food arrives. "I'm from Denmark and we're used to eating at 6 p.m. back home!" As for special preparations, he always carries the same food in his musette, but he'll add warm tea when it's cold, or hydrate with cold water when the warmer weather arrives. When I ask for his advice for beginners in endurance sports, he replies: "I don't think you should think too much. Don't get obsessed with food but appreciate it. I've knocked myself in the head every single time I made a mistake with food. That just killed my morale and happiness. Now, I'm more relaxed with my intake, and I appreciate a good ice cream. I no longer knock myself in the head when I treat myself because I know that the particular ice cream isn't the problem."

I want to know how it felt to win the Amstel Gold Race, as it was great to see one of 'my' riders with such a big win. "I'm not sure that I know. I felt everything and nothing at the same time!" he laughs. "One thing is for sure: the feeling of winning is a blast! It's hard to explain but you'll never get tired of it." So how can people just getting started in the sport enjoy that winning feeling? "Train smart and race easy," he replies. "That's something I've learned from my new coach; that more isn't necessarily better. Feel your body, listen to it, and don't do what others are doing. We're all different." He says that the biggest mistake any new rider can make is to train too much. "It ends up getting way too serious, and you'll stop having fun."

With such great advice from one of the most exciting cyclists to watch, Michael's fun is only just beginning.

Pink Grapefruit, Blueberries, and Dulce de Leche on Oats

Peel the label off of the can of condensed milk. In a large pot filled with room-temperature water over medium heat, completely submerge the can, then slowly bring it to a boil. Reduce the heat to low and simmer for 2-3 hours, depending on how dark and thick you want your dulce de leche to be. Make sure that the can is completely covered in water at all times. Remove it from the heat and set it aside to cool completely before opening. Transfer the dulce de leche into a clean airtight container or piping bag. It will keep in the refrigerator for 2-3 weeks.

With a sharp knife, cut off the grapefruit's top and bottom. Carefully cut off the rind, so that you are only left with grapefruit flesh. Slice the grapefruit into wedges by sliding the knife down next to the membrane on each side. Place the wedges in a bowl, and squeeze any remaining juice within the membrane over them. Halve and pit the plums, then slice them into wedges. Portion the yogurt, oats, blueberries and grapefruit in serving bowls and top them with dots or a drizzle of dulce de leche, then serve.

TIP: Dulce de leche is brilliant in a race food sandwich or as a spread for desserts and cakes.

1 can condensed milk (350 g)

1 large pink grapefruit

2 medium plums

100 g plain Greek yogurt

200 g rolled oats

100 g blueberries

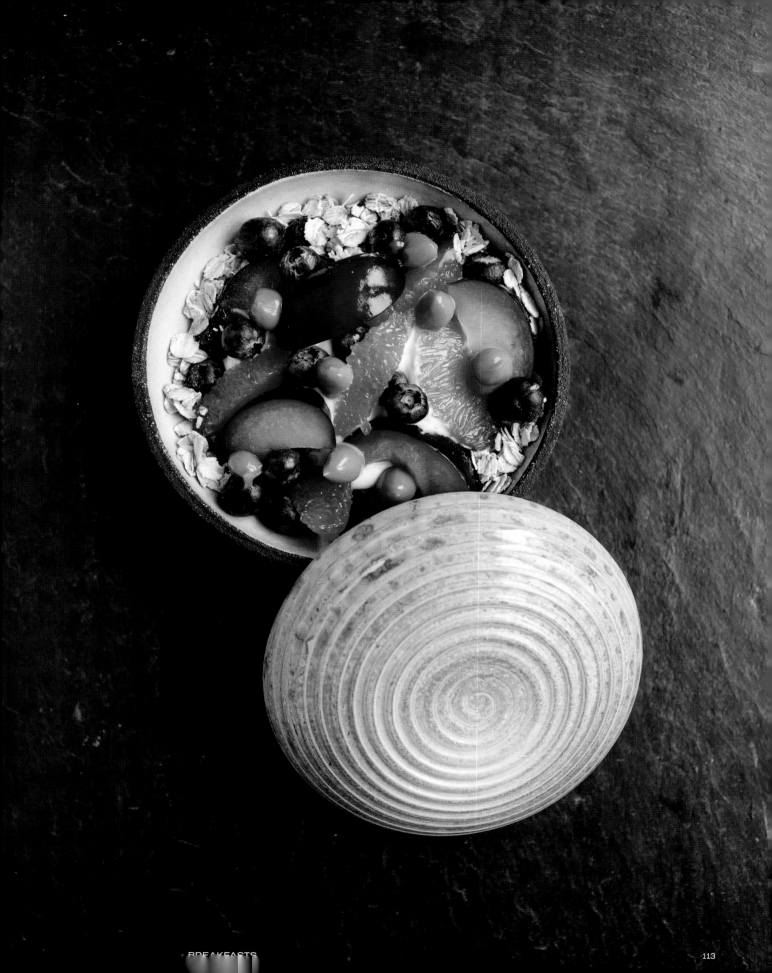

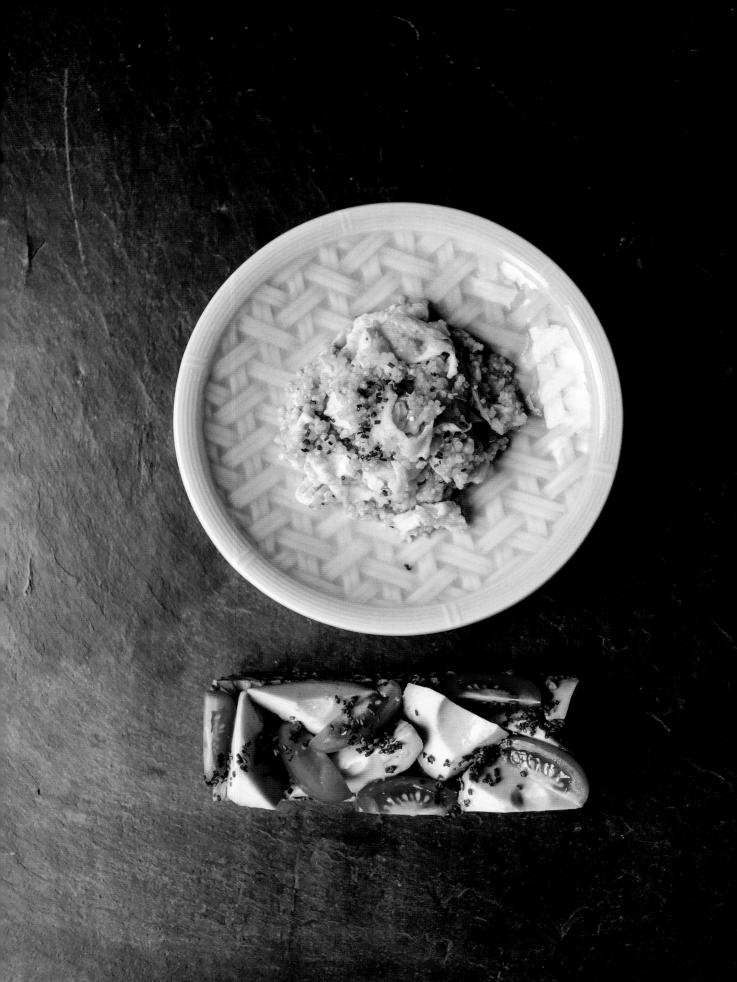

Quinoa Scramble with Tomato and Avocado Toast

Cut the tomatoes into bite-sized pieces. Halve and pit the avocado, scoop the flesh out, and slice it into triangular pieces. Season the tomatoes and avocado with salt, pepper and lemon zest.

Whisk the eggs together in a mixing bowl, then season the mixture with salt and pepper. Heat up a non-stick frying pan over medium heat with the olive oil and warm up the quinoa. Pour the egg mixture onto the pan and scramble it at medium heat with a heatproof rubber spatula. Arrange the tomatoes and avocado on the toasted bread, then plate the quinoa scramble on the side. Top everything with the minced chives.

6 plum tomatoes

1 medium avocado

Salt and pepper, to taste

Zest of 1 lemon

4 whole large eggs

1 tbsp. olive oil

200 g cooked quinoa

2 slices whole grain and seed bread, toasted

1 handful fresh chives, minced

Rösti, Fried Eggs, and Watercress

G D N V

Peel and grate the potatoes. Place the grated potatoes in a cheesecloth or strainer and press vigorously to expel as much moisture as possible. Transfer them into a mixing bowl, then season with salt and pepper.

In a medium-sized frying pan over medium heat, warm 3 tbsp. of olive oil. Tightly pat the shredded potato into a pancake shape in the frying pan and cook for about 5-7 minutes on each side until tender and golden. Transfer the rösti onto a paper towel-lined plate.

Wipe the pan clean with a paper towel. Heat up the remaining olive oil over medium heat. Crack the eggs into the frying pan and fry them for about 2-3 minutes until the egg white has set. Season with salt and pepper. Slice the rösti into 2 or 4 portions, then plate with the eggs and watercress on top.

2 baking potatoes, old

1 yellow onion

4 tbsp. olive oil, divided

2 whole large eggs

50 g watercress, rinsed and dried

Salt and pepper, to taste

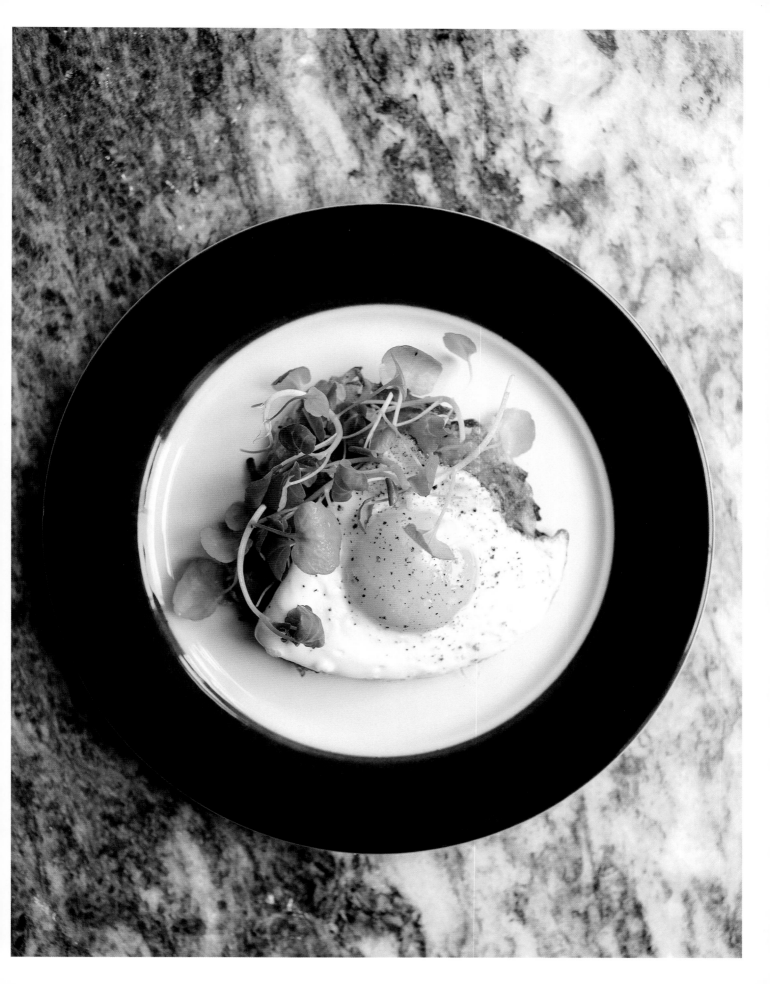

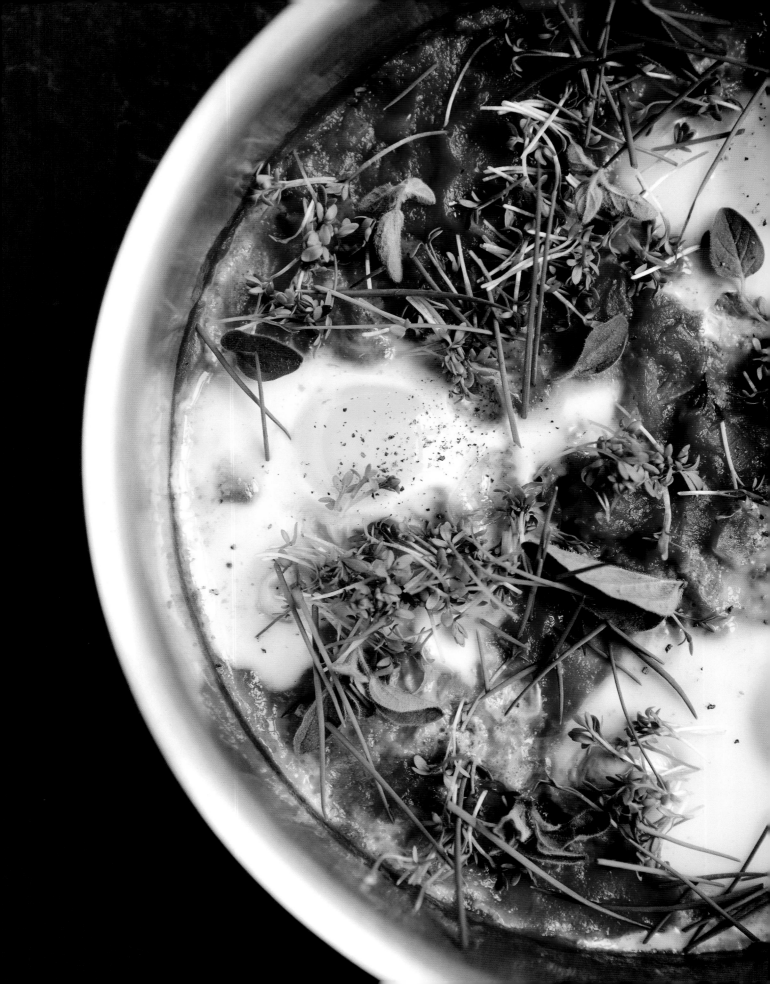

Eggs in Spicy Tomato Sauce (Shakshuka)

Ⓖ Ⓓ Ⓝ Ⓥ

Dice the large tomatoes. Halve the cherry tomatoes, then season them with salt and pepper. Peel the onion and garlic, then slice them thinly.

———

Warm up the olive oil in a thick-bottomed sauté pan. Add the onion, garlic and thyme sprigs. Sauté for about 2 minutes until the onion is tender. Add the diced tomatoes, balsamic vinegar, bay leaves, tomato paste, paprika and chili powder, then bring them to a boil. Season the sauce with salt and pepper to taste.
Reduce the heat to medium-low and simmer for 10-12 minutes until the sauce reduces to a thick consistency. Remove the bay leaves and thyme sprigs, then season with salt, pepper and balsamic vinegar to taste.

———

Reduce the heat to low and make 4 little grooves in the sauce. Crack the eggs into them. Cover and cook for about 5-7 minutes until the egg whites have set but the yolks are still runny.
Remove the pan from the heat. Serve in the pan after topping it with chives, oregano and micro cress with the grilled bread or rice on the side.

� ⅰ – ⅰⅰⅰⅰ

400 g large ripe tomatoes or 1 can

100 g cherry tomatoes

1 medium onion

2 cloves garlic

1 tbsp. olive oil

2 sprigs fresh thyme

3 tbsp. balsamic vinegar + more to taste

2 bay leaves

1 tbsp. tomato paste

1 tsp. smoked paprika

1 pinch chili powder (optional)

4 whole large eggs

Salt and pepper, to taste

Finely chopped fresh chives, to serve

Finely chopped fresh oregano or marjoram, to serve

Finely chopped fresh micro cress, to serve

Grilled bread or cooked rice, to serve

Basic Overnight Chia and Oat Pudding

Combine all the dry ingredients in a bowl. Mix in the wet ingredients, then season with the syrup and salt. Divide into 2 serving bowls and refrigerate overnight with the bowls covered. Serve with the blueberries and lemon zest.

—

TIP: For variations, add shredded carrot, diced apples, cinnamon or nutmeg, and chopped nuts of your choice to make a carrot cake. Or, add 1 tbsp. of cocoa powder and the zest of 1 orange, then top with raspberries to make cocoa and orange with raspberries.

3 tbsp. chia seeds

100 g rolled oats

300 mL almond milk

½ tsp. vanilla extract

200 g Greek yogurt

2–4 tbsp. maple/date syrup

1 pinch salt

100 g blueberries

Zest of ½ lemon

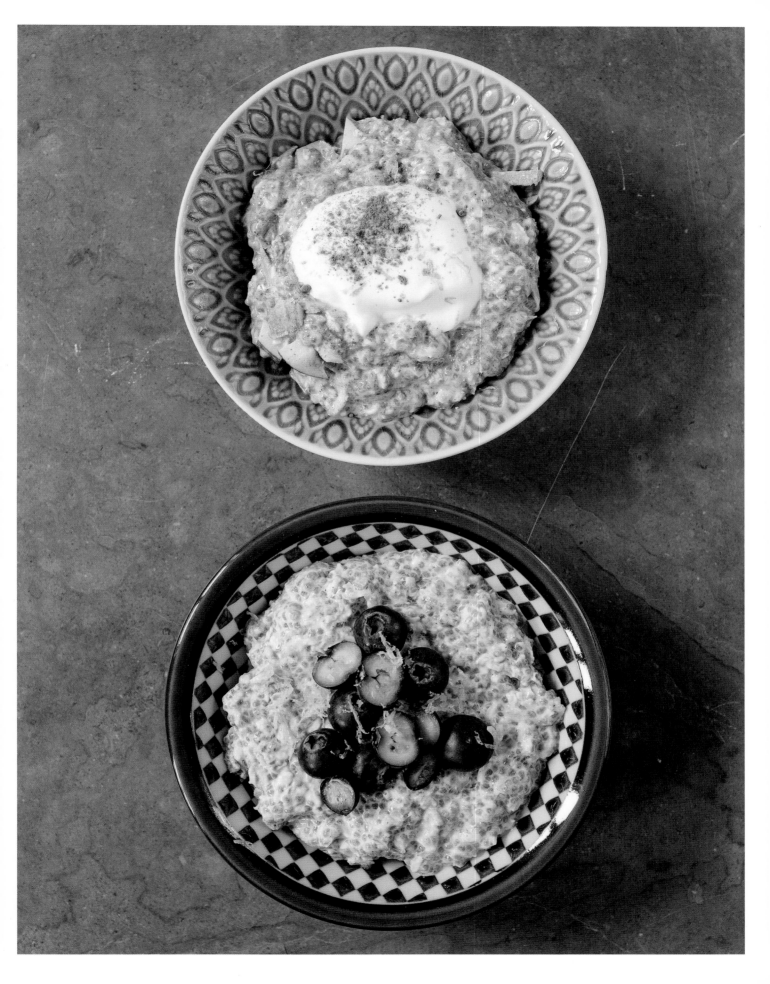

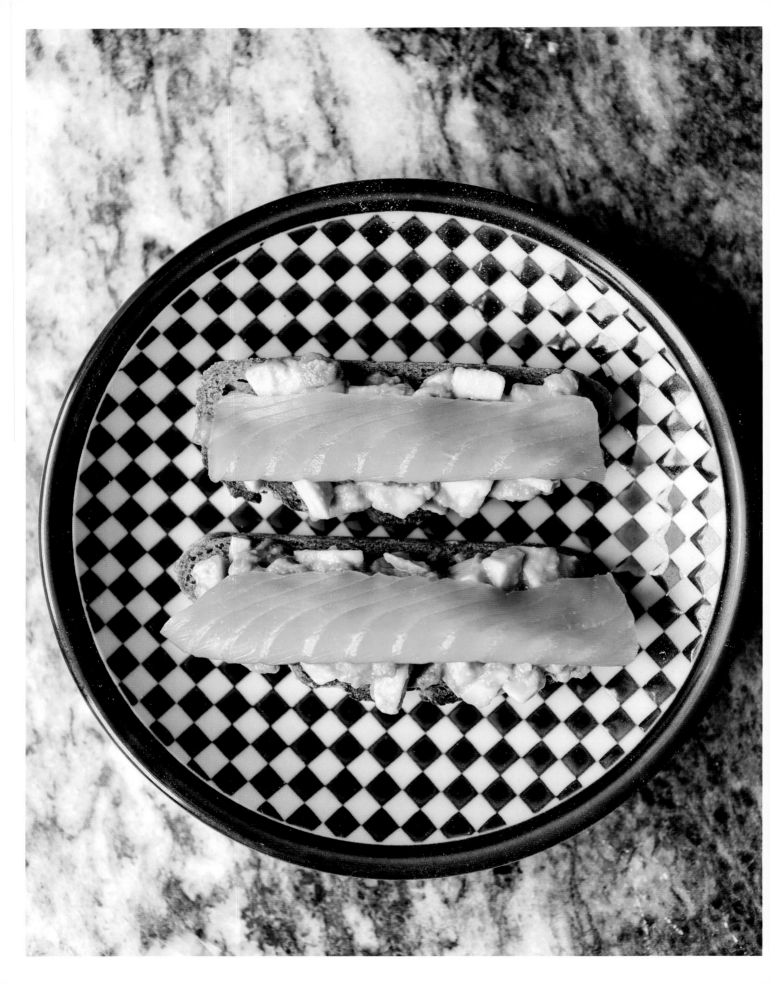

Smoked Salmon
on Avocado Smash Toast

Halve and pit the avocado, then scoop the flesh out into a bowl.
Peel and grate the garlic, then add it into the bowl with the cumin
and lime zest. Crush it all together with a fork or whisk.
Season with salt, pepper and lime juice to taste. Spread the avocado
smash on the bread slices and top with the salmon to serve.

1 medium avocado

1 small clove garlic

1 pinch ground cumin

Zest and juice of 1 lime

2 slices whole grain bread

50 g smoked salmon slices

Salt and pepper, to taste

Green Pea Dip with Spring Veggies

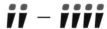

Peel and mince the garlic and shallot finely. Pick and chop the tarragon. In a large sauté pan over medium heat, heat up the olive oil. Add the garlic and shallot to the pan, then sauté for about 2 minutes until the shallot is soft and translucent.

Add the green peas and broth to the pan, then season with salt and pepper to taste. Bring it to a boil and cook for 2 minutes. Remove the pan from the heat. Blend the pea mixture to the desired consistency. Stir the tarragon and lime zest into the purée. Season with salt, pepper and lime juice to taste. Serve the dip with the spring vegetables and grilled bread.

2 cloves garlic

1 shallot

2 tbsp. olive oil

250 g peeled green peas

100 mL water or vegetable broth

500 g raw spring veggies of your choice (e.g. carrots, asparagus, radishes), cut into sticks

½ bunch fresh tarragon

Zest and juice of 1 lime

Grilled bread, to serve

Salt and pepper, to taste

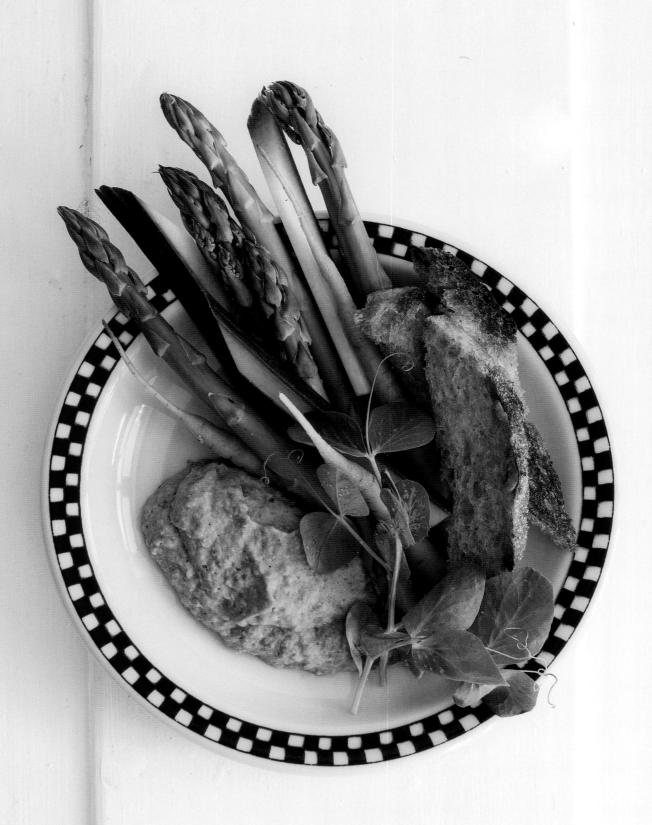

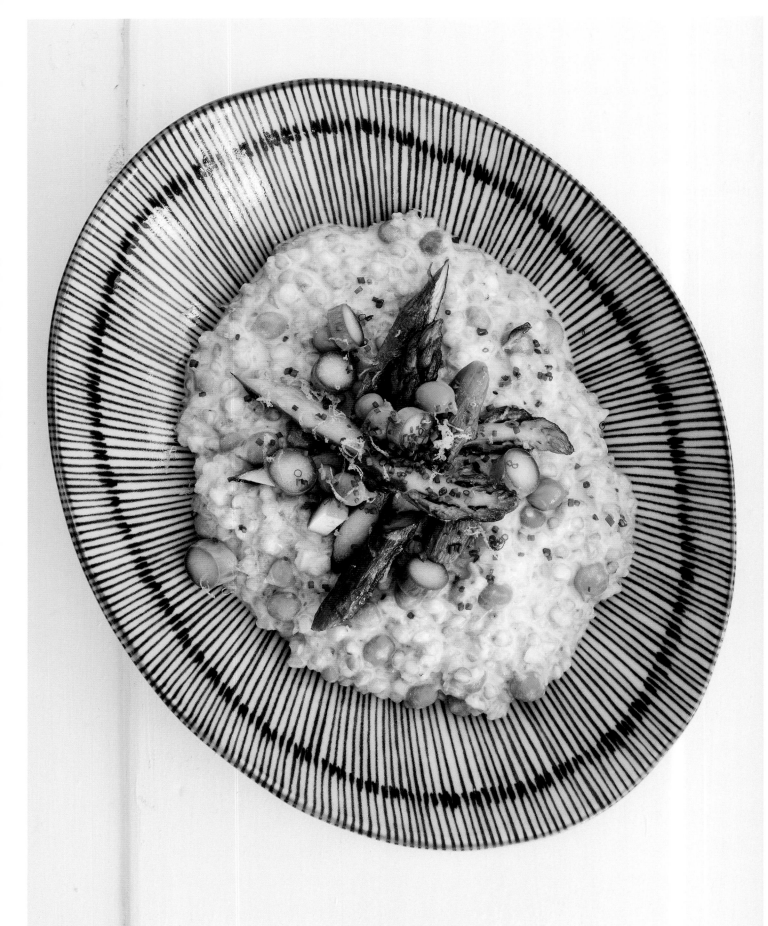

Buckwheat-otto with Asparagus and Peas

Rinse the buckwheat in cold water. In a medium-sized pot over medium heat, cover the buckwheat with water and add ½ tsp. of salt. Bring it to a boil, reduce the heat to low, then simmer covered for 10 minutes until all the liquid has been absorbed. Remove the pot from the heat and set it aside to steep covered for at least 5 minutes. Pour at least 100 mL of excess buckwheat water into a measuring cup and set it aside, then set the pot aside covered.

———

Rinse the asparagus. Break off the bottom parts by holding the asparagus near the end and bending it until it snaps, then discard the ends. Cut the remaining asparagus into bite-sized pieces. Heat up a frying pan with 2 tbsp. of olive oil, sprinkle it with salt, and cook the asparagus over high heat for about 1 minute until they are vivid green and tender with a bite.

———

Heat up the excess buckwheat water and stir it into the warm buckwheat. Fold the yogurt and Parmesan into the warm buckwheat. Season with salt, pepper, lemon zest and juice, then mix in ⅔ of the cooked asparagus.

———

In a small mixing bowl, combine the peas with the remaining asparagus and 2 tbsp. of olive oil, then season with salt and pepper. Place the buckwheat-otto into serving bowls after topping it with the remaining asparagus, peas, lemon zest and minced chives, then serve.

250 g buckwheat

Water, to cover

500 g green asparagus

4 tbsp. olive oil, divided

100 g plain Greek yogurt

100 g freshly grated Parmesan cheese

Zest and juice of 1 lemon

100 g fresh peas, shelled

¼ bunch of chives, minced

Salt and pepper, to taste

Fried Eggs and Lumpfish Roe
with Grilled Asparagus and Avocado

Halve and scoop the avocado flesh out into a mini blender. Add the yogurt and blend until smooth. Season with salt, pepper and lime juice to taste. Set it aside.

———

Rinse the roe in cold water and strain it well, then season with salt, pepper and lime juice. Set it aside. Rinse the asparagus. Break off the bottom parts by holding the asparagus near the end and bending it until it snaps, then discard the ends. Toss the remaining asparagus in 1 tbsp. of olive oil, then season with salt and pepper. Heat up a frying pan over high heat and char the asparagus for 1–2 minutes. Transfer them onto a plate.

———

Wipe the pan clean with a paper towel and fry the eggs in 1 tbsp. of olive oil. Season with salt and pepper. Spread a large spoonful of avocado onto a serving plate with a small pallet knife. Place the asparagus and egg on the avocado, then top them with the roe. Serve with bread or rice on the side.

1 medium avocado

50 g plain Greek yogurt

Juice of 2 limes

100 g lumpfish roe, flying fish roe or salmon eggs

250 g green asparagus

2 tbsp. olive oil, divided

2 whole large eggs

Salt and pepper, to taste

Bread or cooked rice, to serve

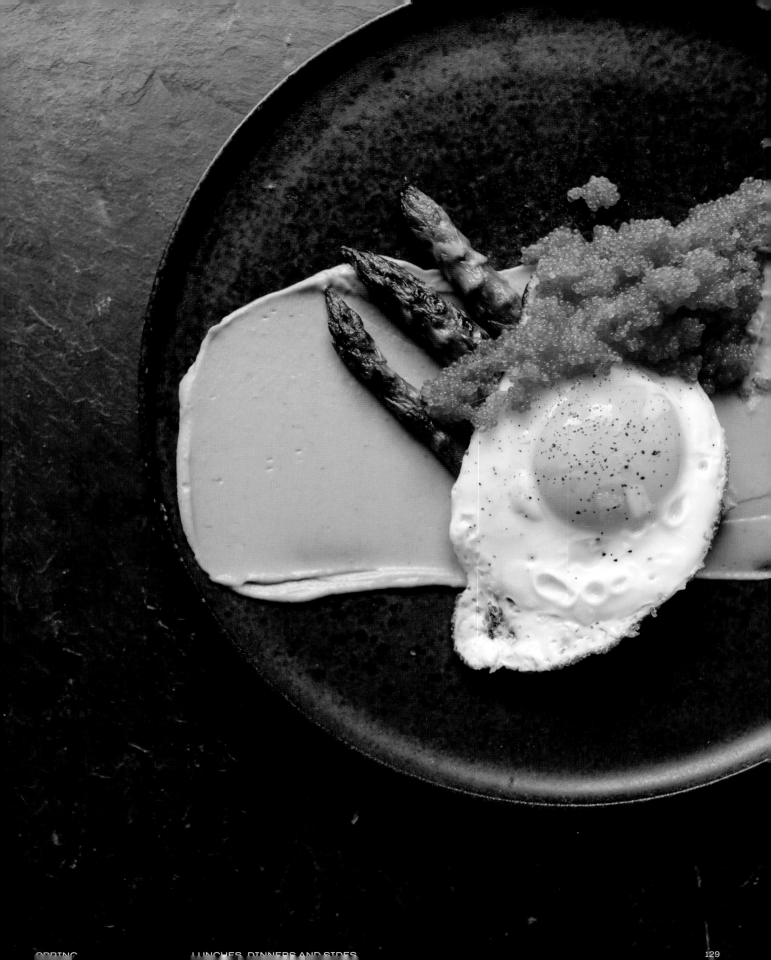

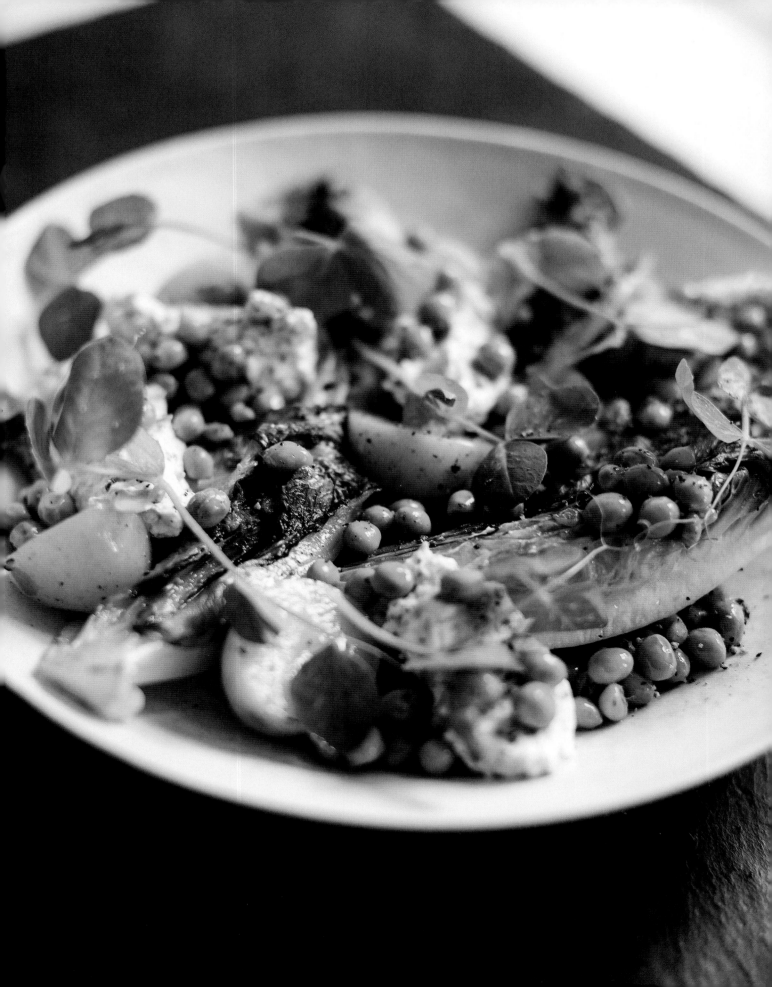

Grilled Little Gem with New Potatoes, Fresh Peas, and Lemon-herb Ricotta

Scrub the potatoes and bring them to a boil in lightly salted water. Turn the heat down to a simmer and cook them under a lid for about 10 minutes. Set the pot aside to steep for 5 minutes, then drain the water. Cool the potatoes down in cold running water. Halve and toss them with 1 tbsp. of olive oil, salt and pepper.

———

Halve the little gem lengthwise. Rinse and spin the water off them. Heat up a frying pan over medium-high heat and sear the cut surfaces until they are caramelized.

———

Mixed the herbs into the ricotta, then season with lemon zest, juice, salt and pepper. On a large serving platter, plate the little gem with the potatoes and peas. Divide the ricotta with a teaspoon and top it with the pea shoots, then serve.

200 g new potatoes

Water, to cover

4 tbsp. olive oil, divided

4 heads little gem lettuce

2 tbsp. finely chopped tarragon

2 tbsp. finely chopped chives

100 g fresh ricotta cheese

Zest and juice of 1 lemon

100 g fresh peas, shelled

Pea shoots, to serve

Salt and pepper, to taste

1-pot Meatballs in Tomato Sauce

Preheat the oven to 180°C/355°F. Soak the oats in the milk. Rinse, pick and chop the mint and parsley. Combine the meat, eggs, garlic, Pecorino and nutmeg, then season with salt and pepper. Add the oats and milk, then mix them by hand until well combined. Set the mixture aside while preparing the sauce.

—

Peel and mince the onions and garlic. Heat up the butter and 1 tbsp. of olive oil in a large pan, then sauté the onions and garlic until the onions are soft and translucent. Add the tomatoes, paste and broth, then bring them to a boil. Season with salt and pepper.

—

With a large spoon or an ice cream scoop, scoop the meatballs into the sauce, drizzle them with olive oil, then season with salt and pepper. Bake for about 25–30 minutes until the meatballs are fully cooked, firm and golden brown. Finish with 3–4 minutes under the grill, then serve topped with fresh tarragon on the spaghetti or grilled bread.

For the meatballs:

100 g rolled oats

80 mL milk

½ bunch fresh mint

½ bunch flat-leaf parsley

400 g ground lamb, beef or veal

2 eggs

2 cloves garlic, crushed

50 g freshly grated Pecorino

½ tsp. freshly grated nutmeg

Salt and pepper, to taste

For the sauce:

2 onions

2 large cloves garlic

2 tbsp. butter

1 tbsp. olive oil + more to cook

2 cans crushed tomatoes (800 g)

100 mL tomato paste

150 mL chicken broth

½ bunch fresh tarragon

Salt and pepper, to taste

Spaghetti or grilled bread, to serve

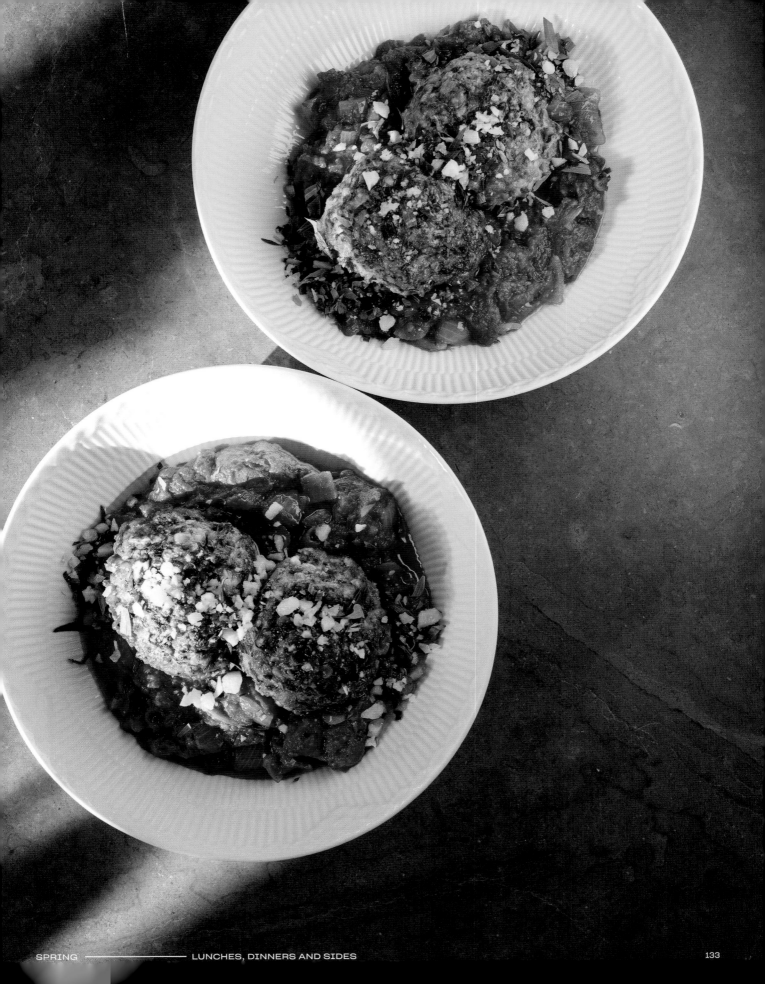

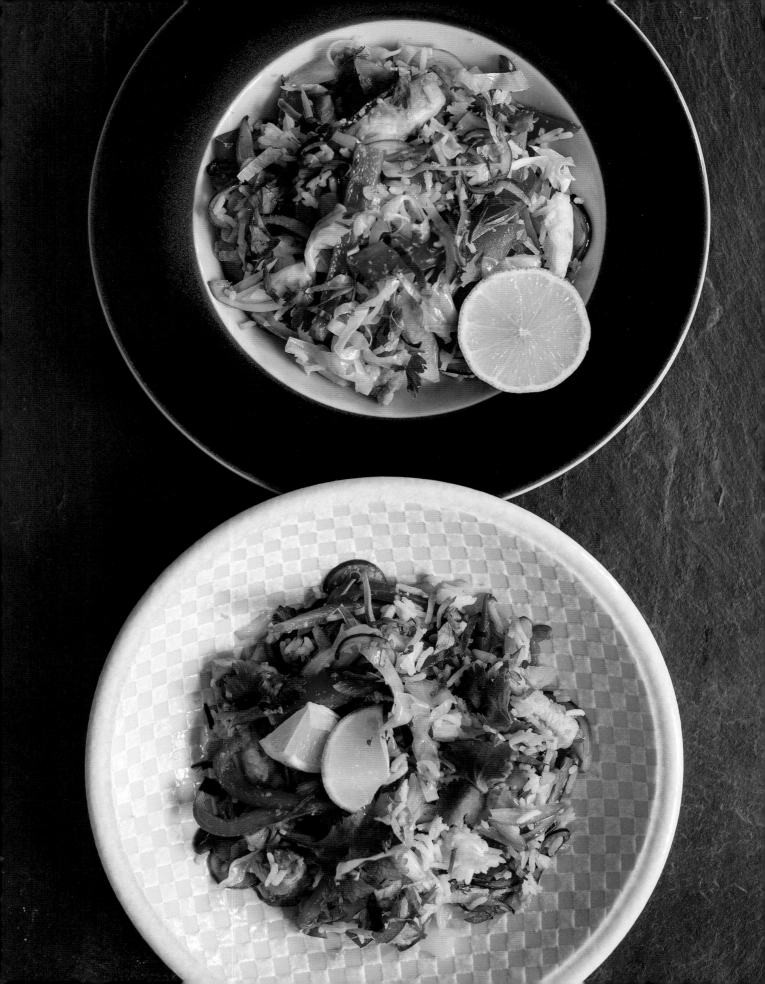

Fried Rice with Pork and Ginger

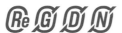

Scrub the ginger clean and peel the garlic. Peel the onions and core the red pepper, then slice them thinly. Shred the cabbage on a Japanese mandolin or using a sharp knife. Mince or finely grate the ginger and garlic, then whisk them into the tamari and 1 tbsp. of olive oil. Trim the pork and slice it into 1 cm × 3 cm strips. Rub the tamari mixture into the pork and set it aside to marinate for at least 10 minutes.

In a large wok or frying pan over high heat, warm the remaining olive oil and add the pork. Cook it through for 2-3 minutes, keeping it juicy and slightly pink. Add and fry the onions and red pepper for about 30 seconds, then add the cabbage and cook for 1 minute. Add the rice and stir until warmed through. Remove the wok from the heat. Season with tamari, lime zest and juice, then serve topped with fresh coriander.

TIP: The pork can be substituted with chicken, tofu, beef, duck, or lamb.

30 g fresh ginger
3 cloves garlic
2 medium red onions
1 medium red pepper
1 pointed cabbage
2 tbsp. tamari + more to taste
2 tbsp. olive oil, divided
200 g filet of pork
400 g cooked rice
Zest and juice of 2 limes
Fresh coriander, picked, to serve

Soba Noodles with Steamed Veggies

Bring 2 large pots of lightly salted water to a boil. Rinse the bok choy and cut it lengthwise into 6 or 8 pieces. Rinse and peel the outer layer of the leeks and cut them into 5 cm-sized pieces.
Rinse the asparagus. Break off the bottom parts by holding the asparagus near the end and bending it until it snaps, then discard the ends.

———

Use plenty of water to cook the soba noodles, as they release a lot of starch. Boil them for about 5 minutes until al dente. Stir the water gently as they boil to prevent them from sticking. Strain them immediately with a colander when done. Rinse the noodles under cold running water until completely chilled. Set them aside to drain completely.

———

Blanch the bok choy into a second pot of boiling water, then plunge them into an ice bath. Place them on a paper towel-lined plate. and sprinkle them with fine salt. Repeat this process with the leeks and asparagus, then discard the boiling water.

———

In a small mixing bowl, make the dipping sauce by whisking the soy sauce and mirin together. Serve the steamed vegetables with the noodles and sauce separately. Dip the vegetables and noodles in the sauce before eating.

———

TIP: This recipe makes a great post-training meal served with a hard-boiled egg or a piece of fish.

1 head bok choy

1 bunch spring leeks

250 g green asparagus

250 g soba noodles

100 mL soy sauce or tamari

50 mL mirin or 1 tbsp. honey mixed with 1 tbsp. water

Fine salt, to taste

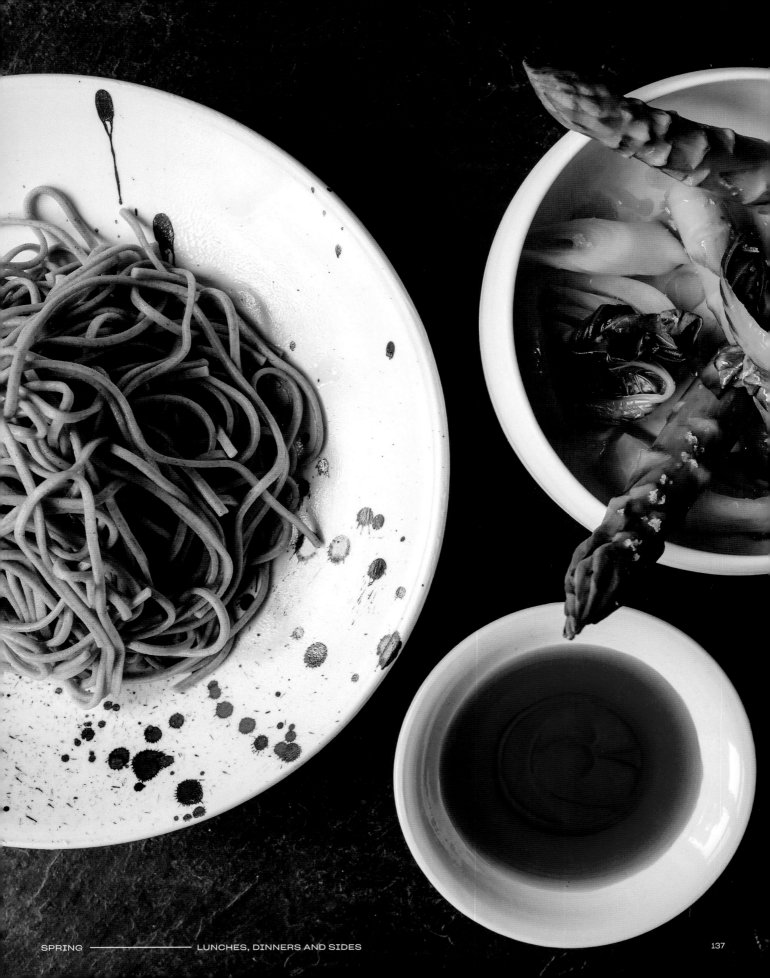

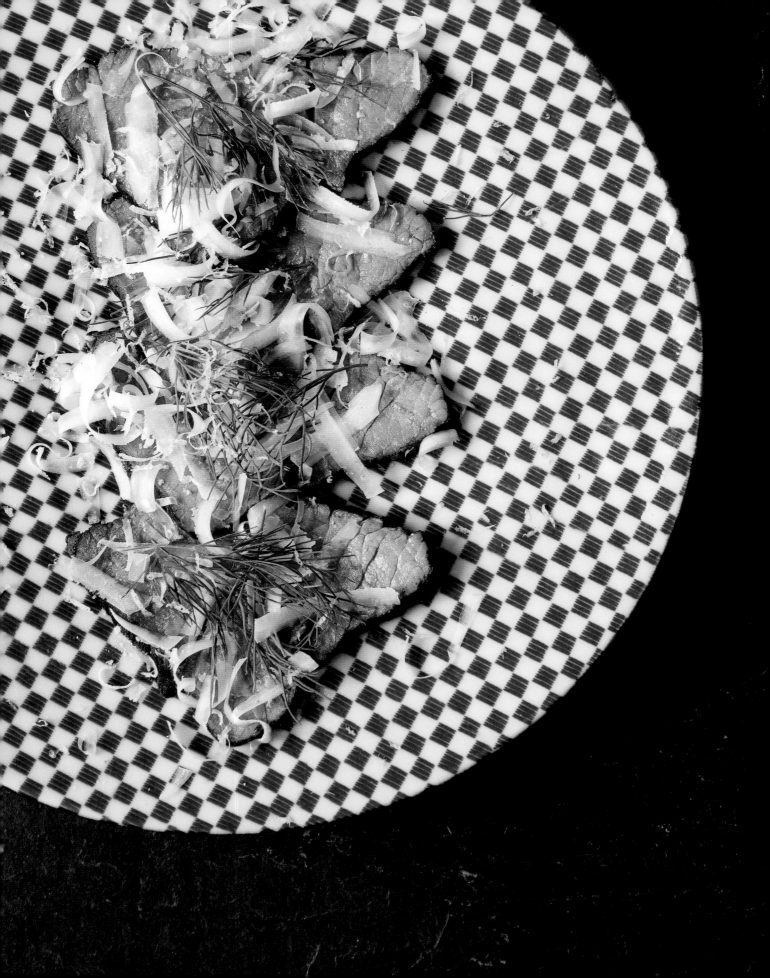

Cold-cut Veal
with Dill, Lemon Zest, and Parmesan

Preheat the oven to 140°C/285°F. To prepare the veal, tie it to roast by cutting a piece of twine about 8 times the length of the veal. Loop the twine around one end of the veal and tie a knot to secure it. Run the twine 2 cm from the knot along the veal. Hold the string down, loop it around the veal, bring it back up to your thumb, and pull it under the twine creating a cross. Repeat this process until you reach the end of the twine, then tie a knot.

———

Rub the veal with 1 tbsp. of olive oil, then season with salt and pepper. Brown the surface on a pan with the remaining olive oil over high heat. Place a meat thermometer in the center of the veal and set the core temperature to:
· 54°C/130°F for red
· 60°C/140°F for medium
· 65°C/150°F for well done

———

Place the veal on a rack on a baking sheet lined with parchment paper, then roast until the desired core temperature is reached. Let the roast rest for 15 minutes before untying and slicing. Season with salt and pepper. Plate the veal slices on a serving platter and top with the Parmesan, dill and lemon zest before serving.

500 g lean veal loin, trimmed of all silver skin

2 tbsp. olive oil

50 g freshly grated Parmesan cheese

1 handful fresh dill

Zest of 1 lemon

Salt and pepper, to taste

Galettes with Goat Cheese, Spinach, and Fried Eggs

Ⓖ Ⓝ Ⓥ

In a large mixing bowl, whisk the water, flour, eggs and salt together. Cover with plastic wrap and refrigerate for at least 30 minutes or overnight.

———

Before cooking, whisk 30 mL of olive oil into the batter. Heat up a non-stick pan over medium–high heat. Pour a ladleful of batter into the pan and swirl the pan around to ensure that the batter spreads evenly. Pour any excess batter back into the bowl. Cook for about 2 minutes on one side and 1 minute on the other side. Transfer the cooked galette onto a plate and keep it covered under tin foil. The first one will most certainly break, but keep going until you get the hang of it. Repeat this process until all the batter is used.

———

Wipe the pan clean with a paper towel and heat it up again over medium heat with ½ tbsp. of olive oil. Add the garlic and sauté for 1 minute until softened. Add the spinach, then season with salt and pepper. Cover the pan with a lid and cook for 30 seconds until it is fully cooked.

———

Heat up another clean pan with 1 tbsp. of olive oil and fry the eggs. Season with salt and pepper. Fill two galettes with spinach and goats cheese. Place 1 egg in the center of each galette and fold the edges over, making a square. Serve immediately with a side salad.

———

TIP: Galettes keep well in the refrigerator in plastic wrap, and they are very handy for a quick breakfast or lunch! To reheat them, cover them with tin foil and pop them into the oven at 180°C/355°F for about 5 minutes until they are warm and soft.

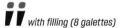
with filling (8 galettes)

750 mL water

250 g buckwheat flour

2 whole large eggs

½ tsp. salt

30 mL olive oil + ½ tbsp. olive oil + 1 tbsp. olive oil, divided

100 g goat or other fresh cheese, crumbled

2 cloves garlic, peeled and thinly sliced

200 g fresh or defrosted spinach

2 eggs, to fry

Side salad, to serve

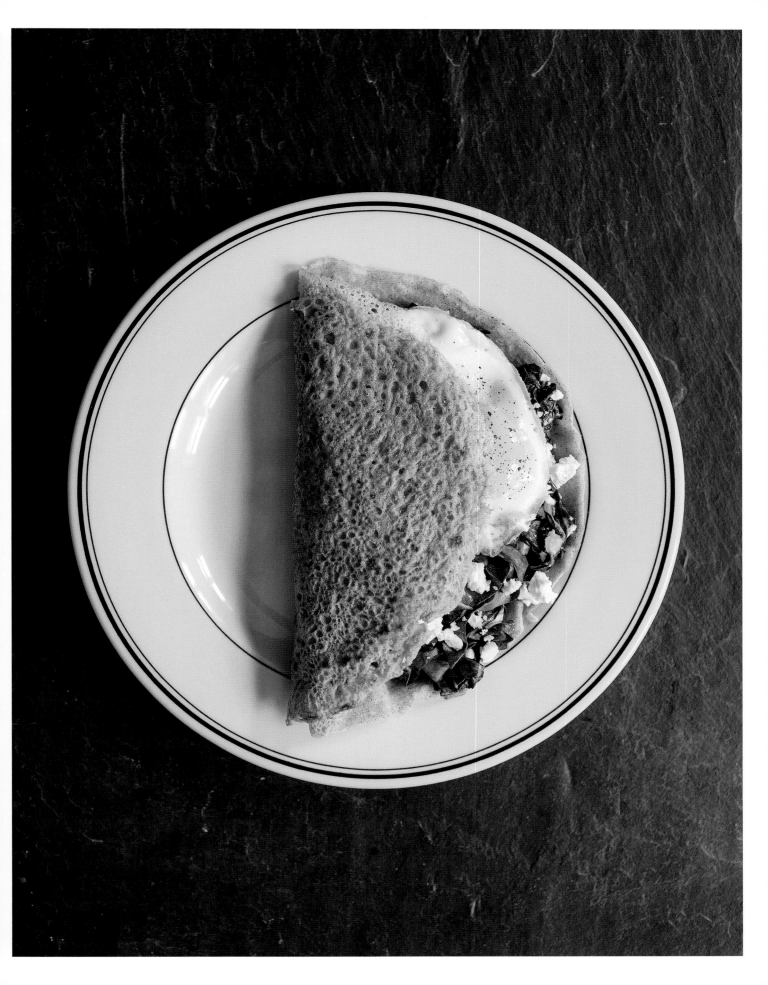

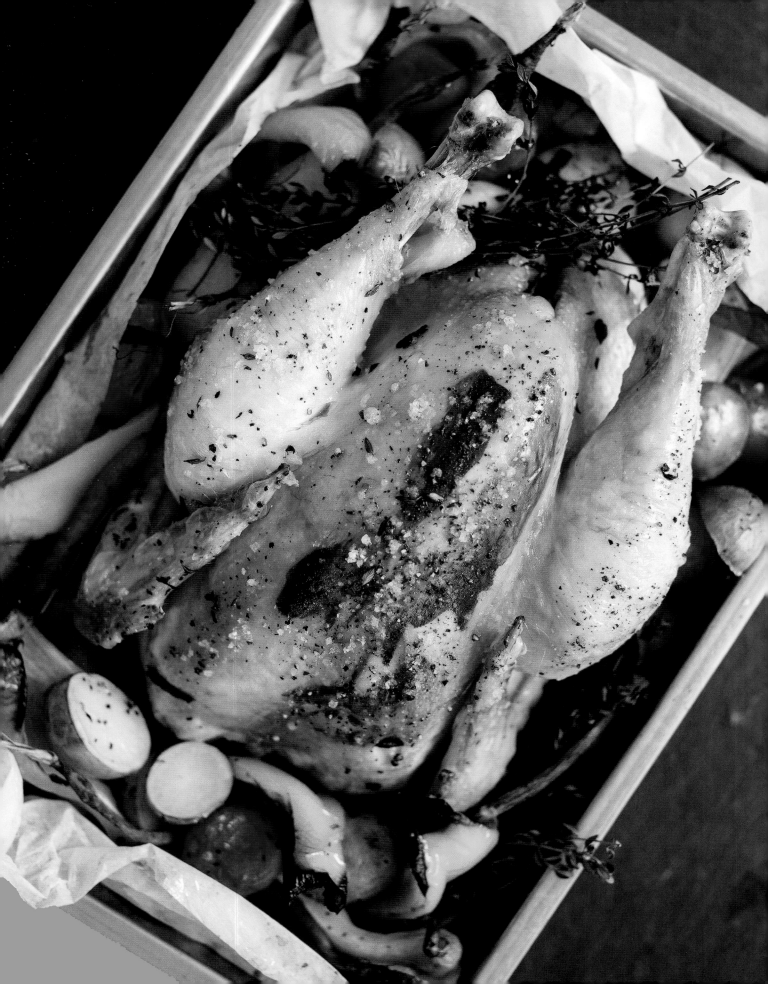

Whole Roasted Chicken with Sage and Garlic on Roasted Veggies

Preheat the oven to 170°C/340°F. Scrub the potatoes and halve them. Rinse all the vegetables and herbs. Halve the tomatoes, core the peppers, then cut them into thick strips. Peel the garlic and slice them thinly. Pick the sage leaves. In a deep roasting pan, combine the potatoes, tomatoes, peppers and thyme. Toss them with 2 tbsp. of olive oil, then season with salt and pepper. Pour the chicken broth over the vegetables.

———

Heat up the butter with the sage leaves and sliced garlic without frying them, then season with salt and pepper. Using your hands, carefully separate the chicken skin from the meat without pulling it off completely. Push the sage butter under the skin all over the chicken, then stretch the skin back into place. Rub the outer skin with the rest of the sage butter, then season with salt and pepper.

———

Place the chicken on top of the vegetables and roast in the oven for 1 hour until the chicken is fully cooked and beautifully roasted. To see if it is fully cooked, prick the thickest part of the chicken leg with a cake tester: the juices should run clear. Let it rest for 15 minutes before carving. Strain the juices from the pan into a sauce pot, bring it to a boil, then season with salt, pepper and apple cider vinegar. Serve the chicken in the pan with the sauce on the side.

1 kg new potatoes

250 g plum tomatoes

1 medium yellow pepper

1 medium red pepper

1 bunch fresh thyme

4 cloves garlic

3 tbsp. olive oil, divided + more as needed

250 mL water or chicken broth

25 g butter, melted

16 sage leaves

1 (1.2 kg) fresh whole chicken, rinsed and patted dry

50 mL apple cider vinegar

Salt and pepper, to taste

Roasted Cucumber
with Pine Nuts, Yogurt, and Coriander

In a large frying pan or grill pan over high heat, heat up the oil. Halve the cucumbers, place them in the frying pan, and char for 2-3 minutes. Remove them from the heat. Slice them diagonally, then season with salt and pepper to taste. Spread the yogurt at the bottom of a deep plate. Top with the cucumbers, pine nuts, coriander and lime zest, then serve.

TIP: To add carbs, cooked quinoa, millet or rice makes an excellent starch base for this dish.

2 tbsp. olive oil

3 medium cucumbers

200 g plain yogurt

50 g pine nuts

1 handful fresh coriander or cilantro

Zest and juice of 1 lime

Salt and pepper, to taste

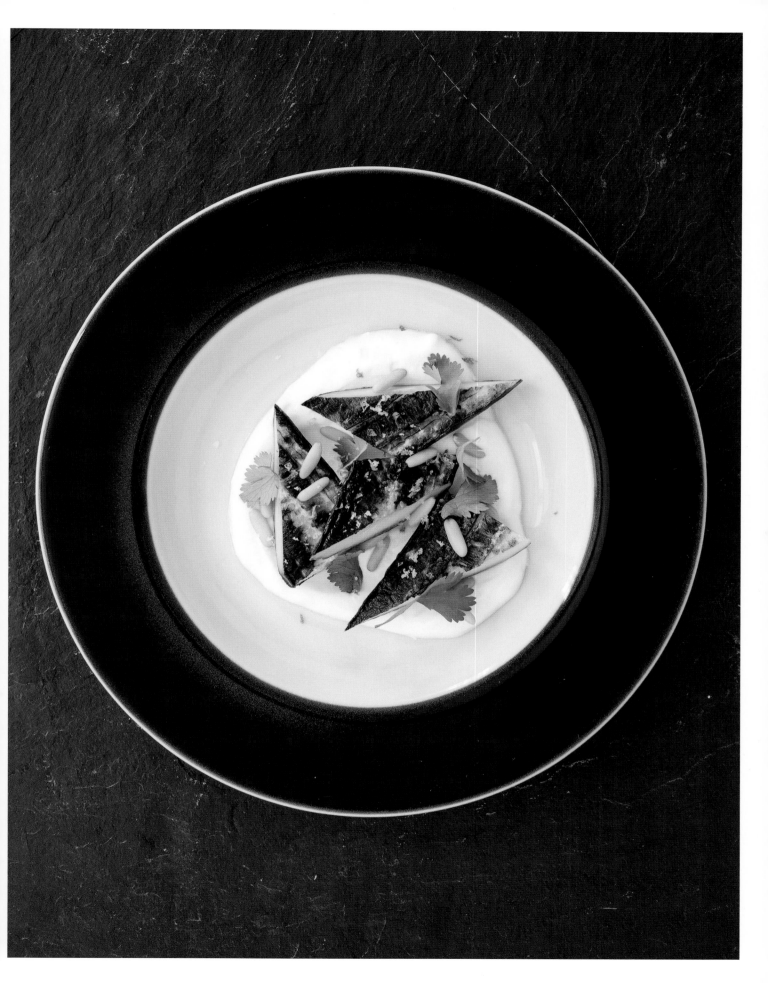

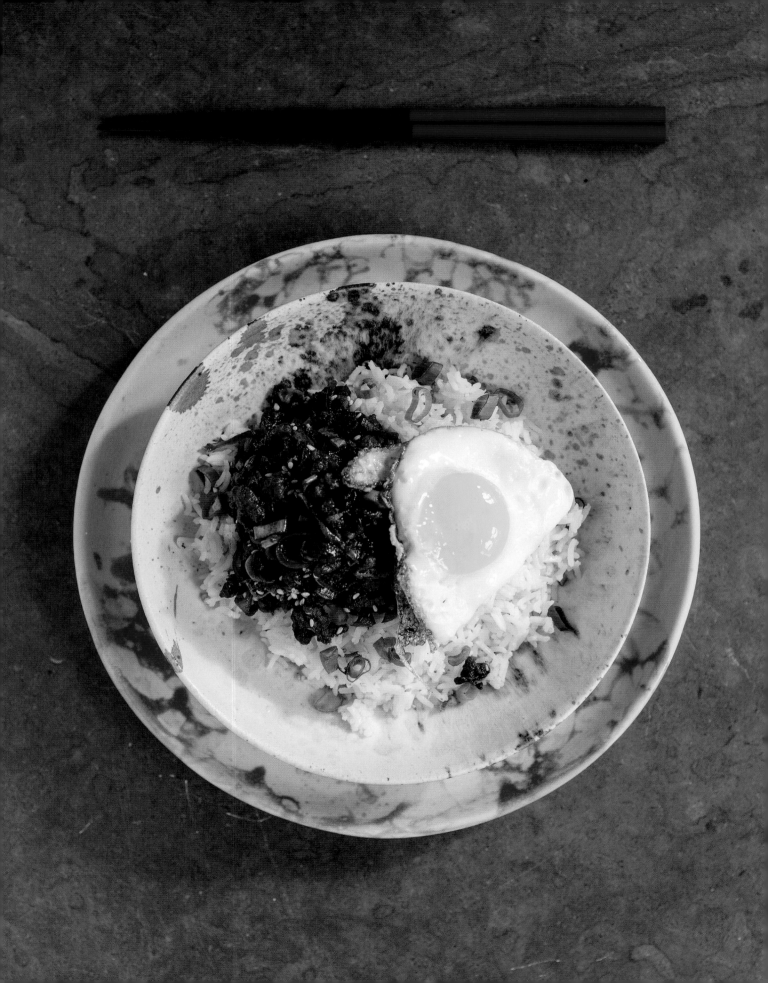

Gyudon or Japanese Beef Bowl with Fried Egg

Bring the rice and water to a boil. Turn the heat down to a simmer, and cook under a lid for 10-12 minutes until all the water has been absorbed. Set the pot aside and let it steep for 12 minutes.

—

Peel and slice the onions and garlic thinly, then mince the garlic. Clean and slice the spring onions thinly. Heat up a large frying pan over medium-high heat, add the olive oil, and brown the beef. Add the onions, garlic and ginger, then sauté until the onions are golden brown and caramelized. Add the soy sauce and mirin, turn down the heat to a simmer, then reduce the liquid down until the meat is beautifully glazed. Add the spring onion and cook for another minute. Season the dish with sesame oil.

—

In a separate pan, fry the eggs and season with salt. Serve the beef and eggs on rice, after sprinkling the toasted sesame on top.

400 g rice + 800 mL water

400 g ground beef

2 onions

4 cloves garlic

1 tbsp. fresh ginger

1 bunch spring onions

2 tbsp. olive oil

50 mL soy sauce or tamari

25 mL mirin or 25 mL water with 2 tbsp. maple/date syrup

1 tbsp. sesame oil

4 eggs

1 tbsp. toasted sesame

Salt, to taste

Cooked rice, to serve

Egg Wrap with Sweet Potato, Avocado, and Grilled Peppers

Re G D N V

Peel and cut the sweet potato into chunks. Boil the chunks with the garlic in unsalted water for about 15-20 minutes until tender. Strain and purée the sweet potato in a blender or mush it up with a fork. Season with salt, pepper lime zest and juice.

Halve and pit the avocado, then scoop the flesh out with a spoon. Slice it and drizzle it with lime juice and salt. Halve and core the peppers. Slice them into thin strips and fry them on a frying pan over medium-high heat in 1 tbsp. of olive oil until dark and tender. Season with salt and cumin.

In a mixing bowl, whisk the eggs, then season with salt and pepper. Transfer the peppers and wipe the pan clean with a paper towel. Return the pan over medium heat and heat up the remaining oil. Pour half the eggs into the pan and swirl the pan so it is coated with a thin layer of egg. Cook for about 1-2 minutes until the layer is set. Flip the egg over and cook for 30 seconds more, then remove it from the heat. Repeat this process with the rest of the mixture for the second wrap. Spread the sweet potato purée over both egg wraps and top with the avocado slices, sautéed peppers, and coriander. Roll up and serve.

1 large sweet potato

1 clove garlic

Zest and juice of 1 lime

1 large avocado

1.5 tbsp. olive oil, divided

1 red pepper

Ground cumin, to taste

4 whole large eggs

1 handful fresh coriander

Salt and pepper, to taste

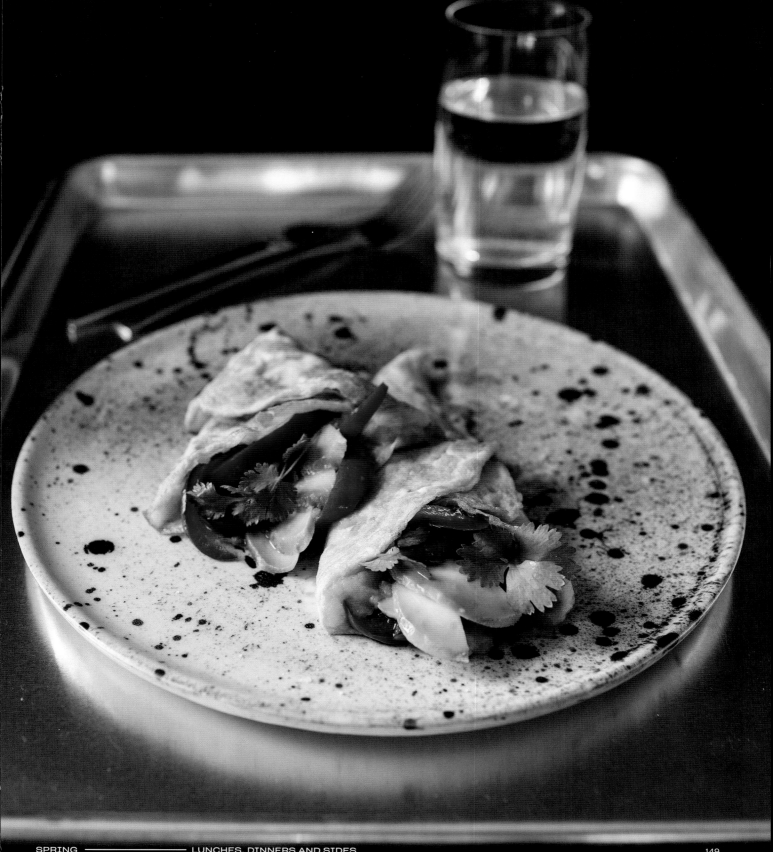

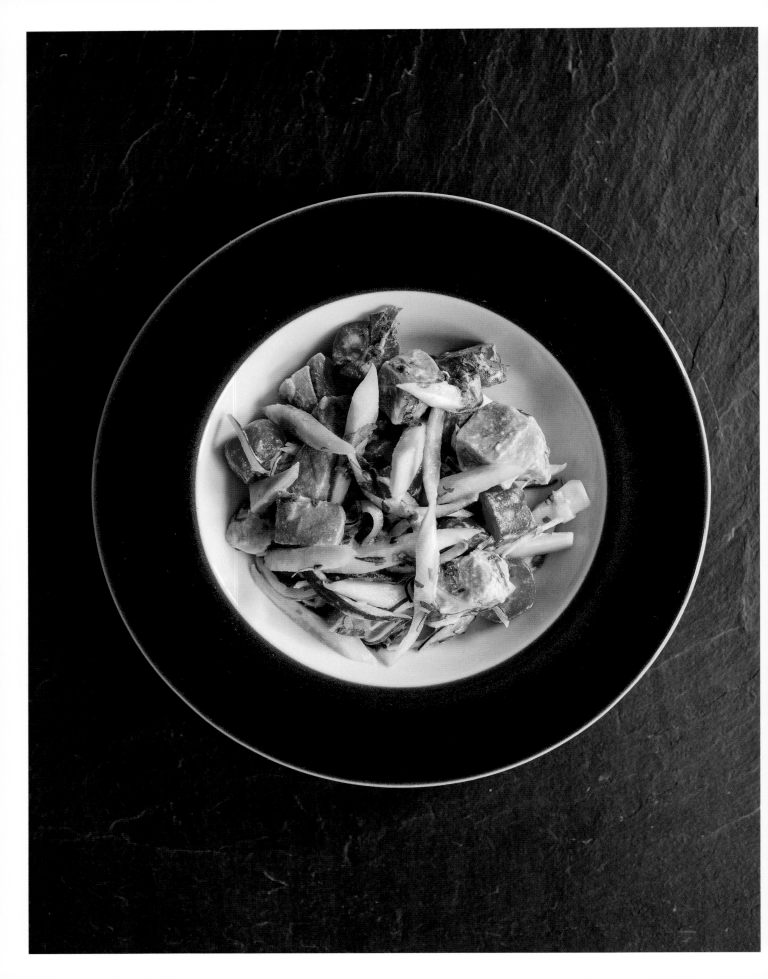

Poisson Cru

Peel and slice the onions, then mix them with the lime zest and juice in a large mixing bowl. Let them marinate with a pinch of salt for at least 2 minutes.

Rinse the tomatoes and halve them. Peel the cucumbers and quarter them lengthwise. Cut out the seeds and discard them. Dice the remaining cucumber flesh. Dice the tuna into 2 cm x 2 cm cubes, then marinate them in the onion mixture for 1 minute. Add the cucumbers, tomatoes and coconut milk, then season with salt, lime zest and juice to taste. Serve cold topped with the fresh coriander.

TIP: To add carbs, serve with cold steamed rice or quinoa.

1 medium red onion

Zest and juice of 2 limes

200 g cherry tomatoes

2 medium cucumbers

200 g fresh tuna

50 mL coconut milk

1 bunch fresh coriander or cilantro

Salt, to taste

Baked Cod, Bok Choy, and Herbs in Vinaigrette

G D N

Preheat the oven to 170°C/335°F. Line a baking sheet with parchment paper. Bring a pot of lightly salted water to a boil. Rinse the bok choy and halve it lengthwise, then slice each half into 3 wedges. Peel off the outer layer of the leeks and split them lengthwise, then rinse them really well under running water. Drop the bok choy into the boiling water and blanch them. Repeat this process with the leeks, but cook the leeks a little bit longer so that they are soft and sweet.

———

Portion the fish into 4 equal-sized pieces and remove any bones and scales. Place the pieces on the prepared sheet and brush them with oil, then season with salt and pepper. Bake for 10–12 minutes until a cake tester slides through the flesh with no resistance. Remove them from the oven.

———

Rinse and mince all the fresh herbs. Peel and mince the shallots, then marinate them in 1 tbsp. of apple cider vinegar. In a small mixing bowl, whisk the remaining apple cider vinegar, mustard, honey and remaining olive oil together. Season with salt and pepper to taste. Add the herbs and shallots into the vinaigrette, then combine well. Top the baked fish with the vinaigrette and serve it with the steamed vegetables.

———

Portion the fish into 4 equal sized pieces and remove any bones and scales. Place the pieces on the prepared baking sheet and brush it with oil and season with salt and black pepper. Bake for 10 to 12 minutes, until a cake tester slides through the flesh with no resistance. Remove from the oven.

———

TIP: To add carbs, serve with crushed new potatoes.

2 bulbs bok choy

2 medium leeks

600 g cod filet, skinned

1 bunch fresh flat-leaf parsley

1 bunch fresh chives

1 bunch fresh tarragon

1 medium shallot

4 tbsp. apple cider vinegar, divided

1 tbsp. Dijon mustard

1 tbsp. honey

6 tbsp. olive oil

Salt and pepper, to serve

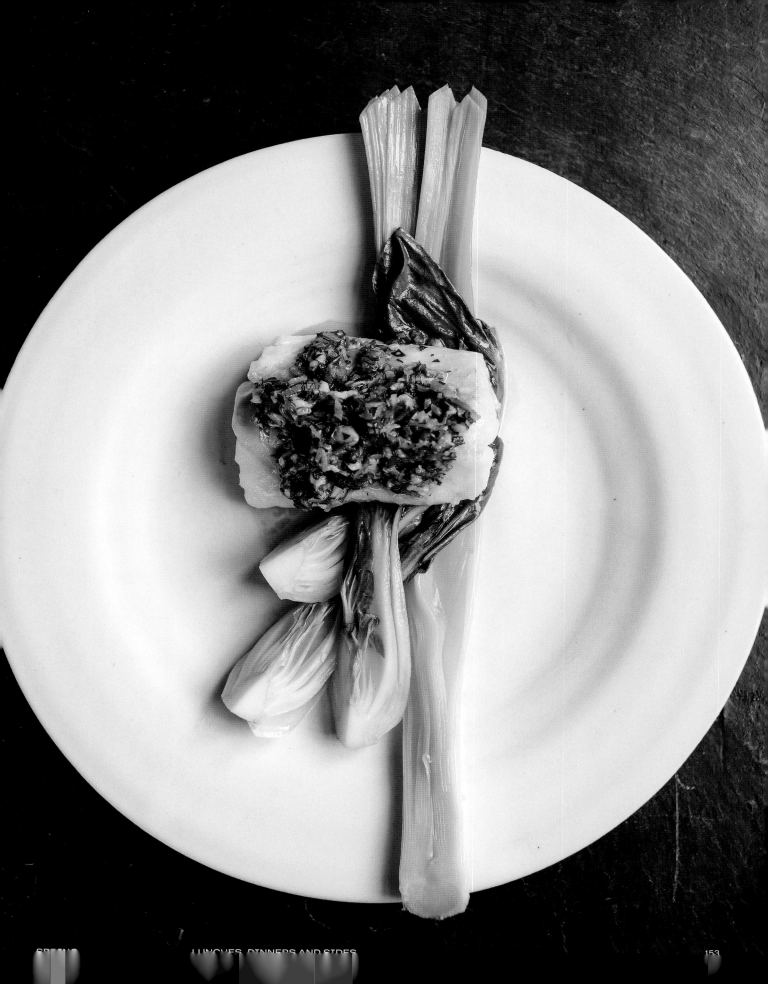

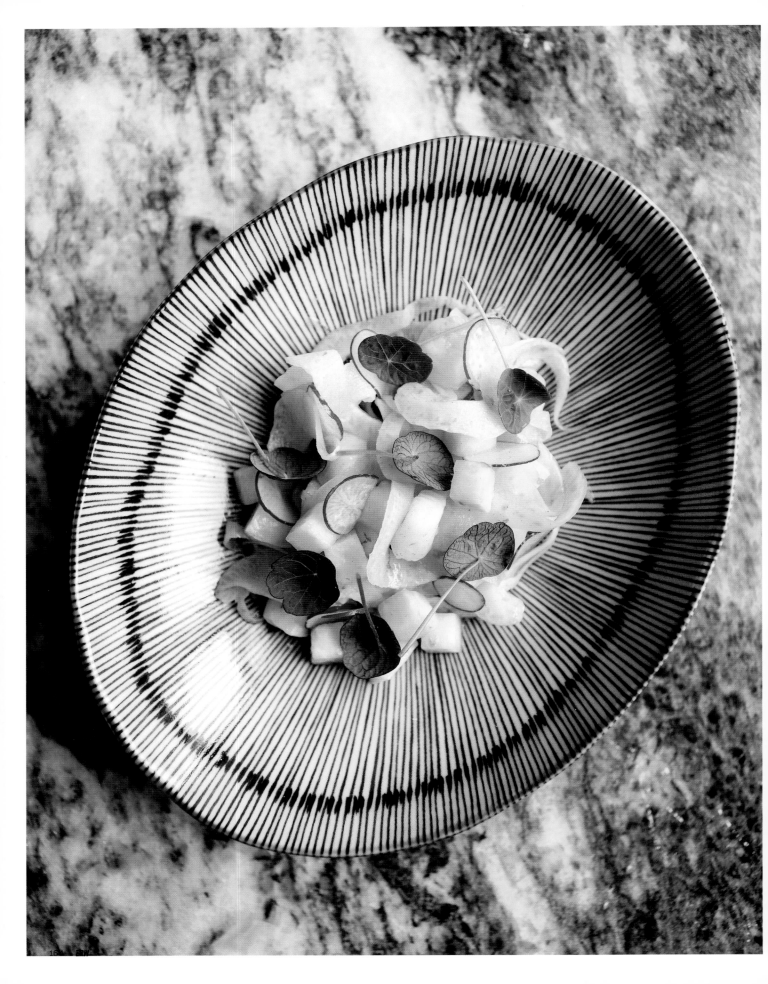

Ceviche with Redfish, Smoked Paprika, and Pineapple

G D N

Remove the bones from the fish and dice it into 1.5 cm–sized cubes. Cut the rind off the pineapple and quarter it. Peel the kohlrabi. Cut the stem off the pineapple and dice both the pineapple and kohlrabi into 1 cm x 1 cm cubes. Rinse the fennel and trim off any brown parts. Slice it thinly on a Japanese mandolin and submerge the pieces in cold water with the juice of ½ a lime.

———

Mix the fish with the remaining lime zest and juice in a mixing bowl, then sprinkle it with salt. Let the fish marinate for about 2 minutes. Add the pineapple, fennel, kohlrabi, olive oil and paprika into the bowl, then combine well. Season with salt and more paprika to taste. Serve topped with the nasturtium or watercress.

———

TIP: To add carbs, serve with steamed rice.

400 g redfish filets, skinned

½ fresh pineapple

1 kohlrabi

1 fennel bulb

Zest and juice of 2 limes

2 tbsp. olive oil

1 pinch smoked paprika + more to taste

1 handful fresh nasturtium leaves or watercress

Baked BBQ Chicken

Preheat the oven to 175°C/335°F. To make the marinade, peel and shred the garlic finely into a mixing bowl. Combine the olive oil, tomato paste, apple cider vinegar, honey, sesame seeds, paprika, cumin and chili pepper. Season with salt and pepper to taste, then stir until well combined.

———

Coat the chicken legs completely in the marinade and transfer them onto a baking dish. Pour the remaining marinade over the chicken. Roast for 35–40 minutes until the chicken is caramelized and fully cooked. Spoon the marinade over the chicken occasionally as it roasts. Serve hot after toping with fresh coriander or spring onions.

———

Tip: To add carbs, serve with roasted potatoes or steamed white rice. To maximize the flavor, marinate the chicken the night before and refrigerate them in a sealed plastic bag.

2 cloves garlic, peeled and minced

50 mL olive oil

50 g tomato paste

30 mL apple cider vinegar

30 mL honey

2 tbsp. white sesame seeds

1 tablespoon smoked paprika

1 tsp. ground cumin

1 medium chili pepper (optional)

Salt and pepper, to taste

4 fresh chicken legs

1 bunch fresh coriander or spring onions, picked, to serve

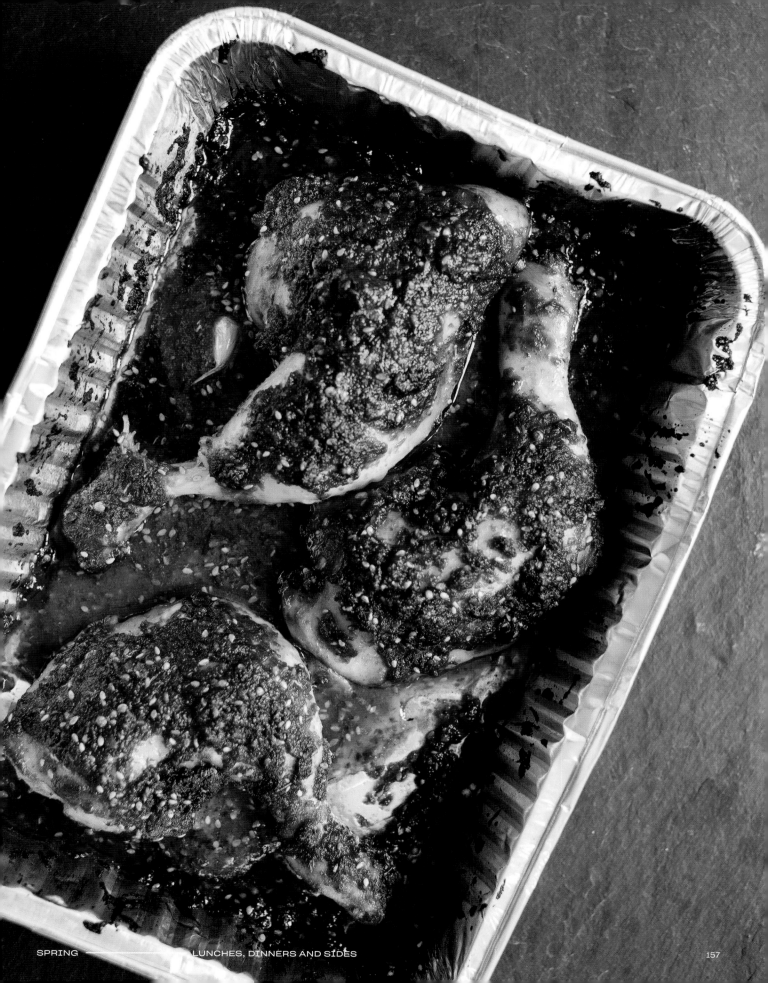

Sprouting

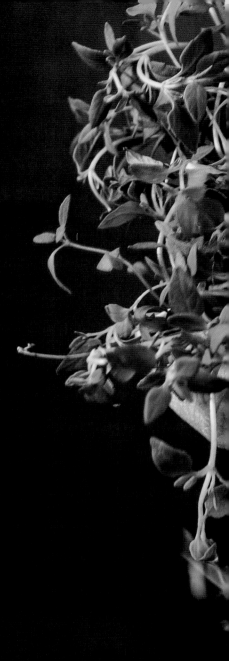

Our bodies are said to recognize sprouts of grains and legumes as vegetables instead of starches. The sprouting process turns starchy grains and legumes into living plants with nutrients that are better for our digestive systems.

Why sprout?

Sprouted grains are easily digestible nutrient bombs that can be eaten all year round in salads, soups, snacks, and more. These little mineral- and vitamin-packed seeds will also brighten your winter meals and keep you well nourished throughout the dark and cold months.

How to sprout:

When a seed is soaked in water under the right conditions, it will start to sprout. However, there are a few simple rules that must be followed to ensure clean and healthy sprouts. Always use a see-through container with a perforated lid at room temperature, and keep it out of the sunlight.

—

Step 1 - Soaking
Rinse the sprouts and soak 1 part seeds to 2-3 parts water. Most seeds need 8-12 hours before they are fully soaked. Remove all floating bits and pieces from the water surface after soaking.

—

Step 2 - Rinsing
Drain the soaked seeds and rinse them well under cold running water at the highest pressure to oxygenate and clean the seeds. The seeds should be rinsed 2-3 times a day to keep their moisture balance intact.

—

Step 3 - Draining
Get as much water drained from the sprouts after each rinse. A good way to do this is to use a salad spinner. Repeat steps 2 and 3 as many times as needed, depending on the grain. The sprouts can be refrigerated in a sealed container for 4-6 weeks. Serve them raw or after gently heating them up.

—

TIP: Always choose organic seeds and grains to ensure the highest-quality outcome. Taste your sprouts after soaking and rinsing them to find the perfect time to harvest them.

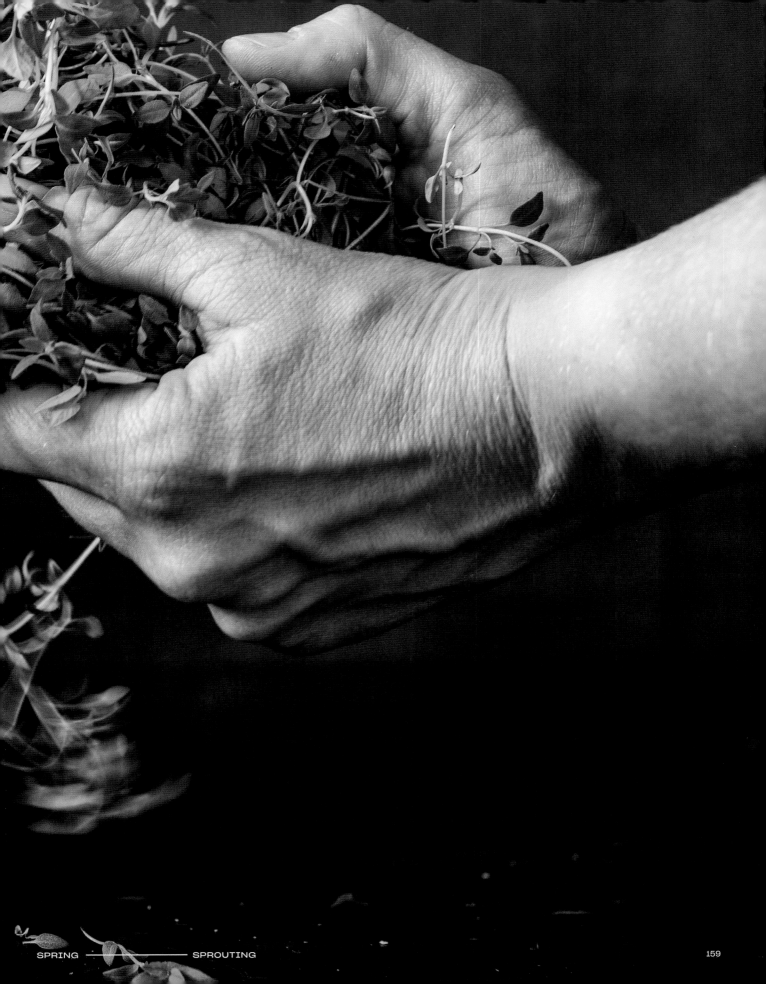

Pumpkin Sprouts

—

Soak 1–4 hours
Rinse 2 times a day
Ready in 1–2 days, or grow until desired size

Sunflower Sprouts

—

Soak 1–2 hours
Rinse 2 times a day
Ready in 1–2 days, or grow until desired size

Buckwheat Groats

—

Soak 30 minutes
Rinse 2 times a day really well, to get all the starch out
Ready in 1–3 days

Yellow Pea Sprouts

—

Soak 8–12 hours
Rinse 2-3 times a day
Ready in 2–3 days

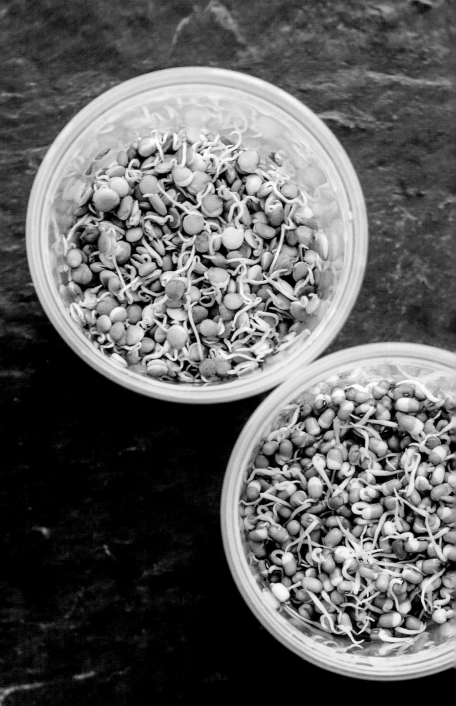

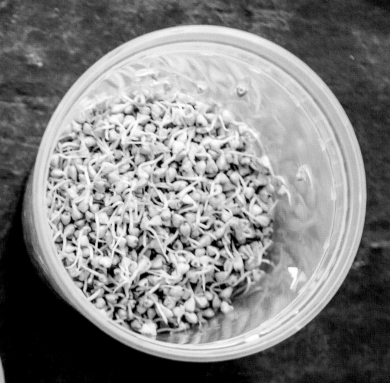

Mung Bean Sprouts

—

Soak 8–12 hours
Rinse 2–3 times a day
Ready in 2–5 days

Green Lentil Sprouts

—

Soak 8–12 hours
Rinse 2–3 times a day
Ready in 2–3 days

Chickpea Sprouts

—

Soak 12 hours
Rinse 2–3 times a day
Ready in 3–5 days

Sprouted Almonds

—

Soak for 4–12 hours
Rinse 2 times a day
Ready in 1–3 days (these bulk up instead of
sprout)

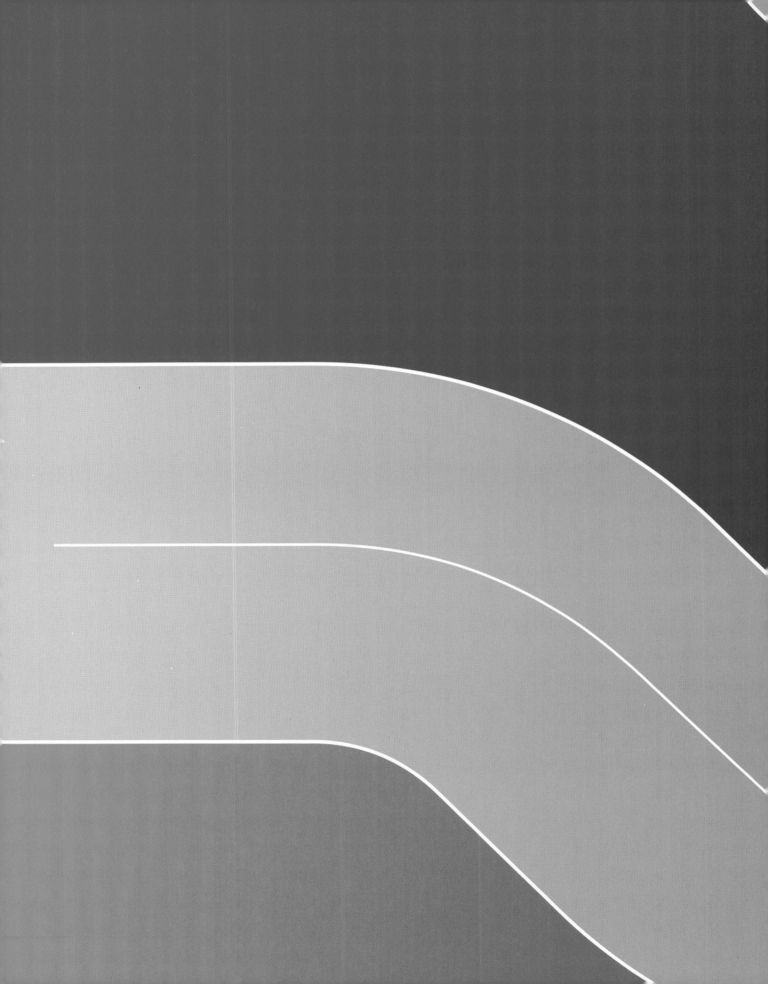

ERW
SUMMER

Summer Breakfasts

Summer Lunches, Dinners and Sides

SUMMER: HIGH SEASON

Long days, sunny training, and racing adventures - in summer, the body is fighting fit and needs the right nutrition to keep it going through the intensity. Heat will take a toll, not only on your ability to recover and sleep, but also on your total body hydration and gut microbiome.

In this section, you will find recipes that support lean mass reparation, keep your body fat down and hydration levels up, as well as ensure that your gut flora stays happy. Meals for summer should be high in carbohydrates (40%-45%), low in fats, and contain moderate amounts of protein.

Eat Race Win! Keywords for Summer

- Grilled foods

- Polenta

- Cold foods that get their heat from spices, their sweetness from maple/date syrup and honey, and their fiber and pectin from fruits

- Lots of citrus fruits

- Breakfasts with carbs and proteins that are low in fats and nut butters

- Lunches that are carb-dense and stocked with lean and light protein, to act as recovery meals

- Dinners with lean red meats, cold-pressed fats, nut butters, and foods high on the GI list

- For racing foods, polenta and rice bars, and caffeine punch balls containing cashews, almonds, dates, cocoa powder, espressopowder, and cocoa nibs

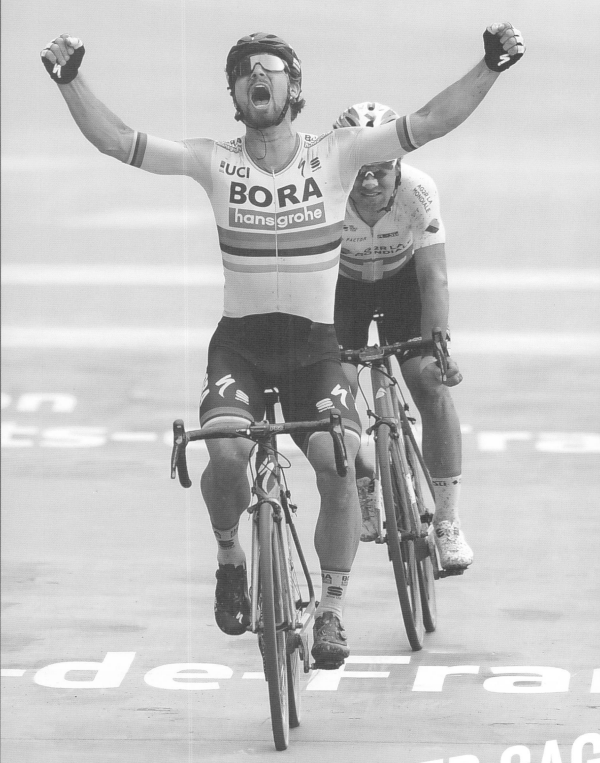

PETER SAGAN

Born — 26 January 1990
Origin — Slovakia

"A well-balanced diet is a must to reach peak performance."

Peter Sagan has had an amazing career full of firsts. He was the first rider to win three world champion rainbow jerseys in a row, and the first Slovak rider to win the Tour of Flanders as well as the Paris-Roubaix; but he could not have done it without the right fuel. "A car does not work if it has no fuel, or if you fill it up with water instead of diesel or petrol," he tells me. "It's the same for a rider: if I don't fuel my body or fuel it with something other than what I need, I'll definitely not reach my desired performance." Can he feel the difference in his performance when he eats the right food? "Absolutely," he says. "A well-balanced diet is a must in order to reach peak performance."

Peter considers himself lucky. Unlike the specialist climbers who depend on a high power-to-weight ratio to conquer the fearsome climbs of the Alps and the Dolomites, he doesn't have to watch his weight that much. "I don't think I'm the kind of rider who has to watch every calorie!" he laughs. "Of course, I have certain limitations, but these are more related to the diversity of my diet." So what works best for a world champion before an important race? "Definitely a good sleep, staying stress-free, and eating an appropriate dinner as well as an energy-filled breakfast on race day." For the best recovery: "We were told that pure glucose straight after a race helps the muscles to recover, but I think a good sleep is best!"

So what does Peter typically eat before a big performance? "For dinner, I normally eat meat with some carbs like potatoes, rice, pasta, and salad. In the morning, it's mostly sweet stuff for energy like cereals, bread, jam, coffee, and sometimes even rice or pasta, depending on the race. I try to skip refined sugar and sweeten my food with alternate sugars, like syrup made from topinambur (Jerusalem artichoke), which is a new product for our team."

I ask him if he'd consider tweaking his diet, but he mentions that it works just fine for him as it is - although he has started to eat more fish. "I wasn't a big fan until Hannah cooked it for me, and it has to be cooked that way all the time now," he laughs. It's all part of the well-balanced diet that he follows all-year round, while eating smaller amounts to match his lower energy requirements. "I eat what I have to eat," he says simply.

Peter started his run of world championship victories in 2015 with the Tinkoff team, and the first rainbow jersey remains the highlight of his career. "Every victory delights me, but the most precious one is the first world championship." Holding off a charging peloton, Peter won his first title in a thrilling finish on the streets of Richmond, U.S.A. It was a great result after a season in which he'd been frequently criticised for finishing second, telling his critics he was happy just to ride his bike and put on a show. How did he feel when he crossed the finish line? "I don't remember," he says. "These emotions are so special and one-of-a-kind that you can only feel them in that specific moment."

So how can an amateur rider become the next Peter Sagan? What advice does he have for a new rider with big ambitions? "I'd say the one thing to avoid is changing your diet completely," he tells me. "If your body has been used to the same kind of food for 20 or so years, it's a big stress to start eating something completely different." He is thoughtful in his recommendations for riders who want to eat properly and be full of energy: "It's hard to say, because what works for me might not necessarily work for somebody else. I think it would be best to follow a balanced diet and get to know what works best for your own body."

Eat healthily, ride fast, and keep winning - that's the Peter Sagan formula for success.

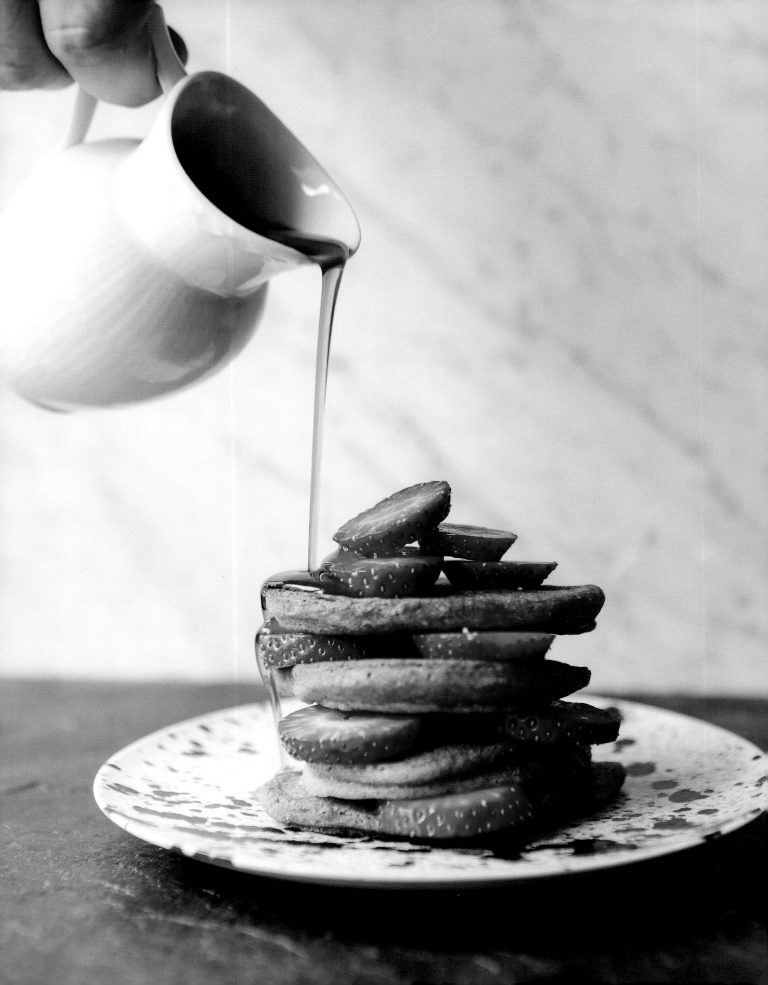

Banana-oat Pancakes
with Strawberries and Maple Syrup

G D N V

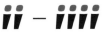

Blend the oats into flour in a food processor or blender. Mash the bananas in a large mixing bowl and combine them well with the oat flour, eggs, cinnamon and salt. Heat up a non-stick pan with ½ tbsp. of oil and add 3 spoons of batter from the mixing bowl. Fry for 1.5 minutes on one side, then flip over and cook for another minute until set and golden brown. Serve the pancakes warm after topping with the strawberries and maple syrup.

80 g rolled oats

3 ripe bananas

4 eggs

1 pinch cinnamon

1 pinch salt

Oil, to cook

400 g strawberries, diced

Maple syrup, to serve

Cinnamon-egg Crepe with Fruit and Rice

Re G N V

Rinse and dry the orange. With a sharp knife, cut off the top and bottom. Carefully cut off the rind, so you are only left with the orange flesh. Slice it into wedges by sliding the knife down next to the membrane on each side. Place the wedges in a bowl, and squeeze any remaining juice within the membrane over them.

———

Hold the pomegranate half face-down in the palm of your hand over a bowl of water. Hit the top of the pomegranate with the back of a wooden spoon and let the arils fall out into the water. Remove the white membrane and strain the arils. Transfer them into the bowl containing the orange wedges.

———

Slice 2 sides of the mango as close to the stone as possible. Discard the stone and cut a grid into the flesh of each side of the mango. Flip the mango halves inside out and then carefully slice the pieces of mango away from the skin. Place them into the bowl containing the orange wedges and pomegranate arils. Add the rice, blueberries and yogurt into the bowl and stir until well combined. Season the mixture with honey to taste. In another bowl, whisk the eggs, cinnamon and salt together. Season with honey to taste.

———

In a large non-stick pan over medium heat, heat up the olive oil. Pour a ladleful of the egg mixture into the pan. Turn the pan until the mixture is thinly spread, cook for 1 minute until the crepe is set, then flip it over and cook for ½ a minute. Remove it from the pan onto a plate and repeat this process until all the mixture has been used. Serve by wrapping the fruit and rice mixture with the crepe.

1 medium orange

½ pomegranate

1 medium mango

400 g cooked rice

50 g fresh blueberries

2–4 tbsp. plain Greek yogurt

Honey, to taste

4 whole large eggs

1 pinch ground cinnamon

Salt, to taste

1 tsp. olive oil

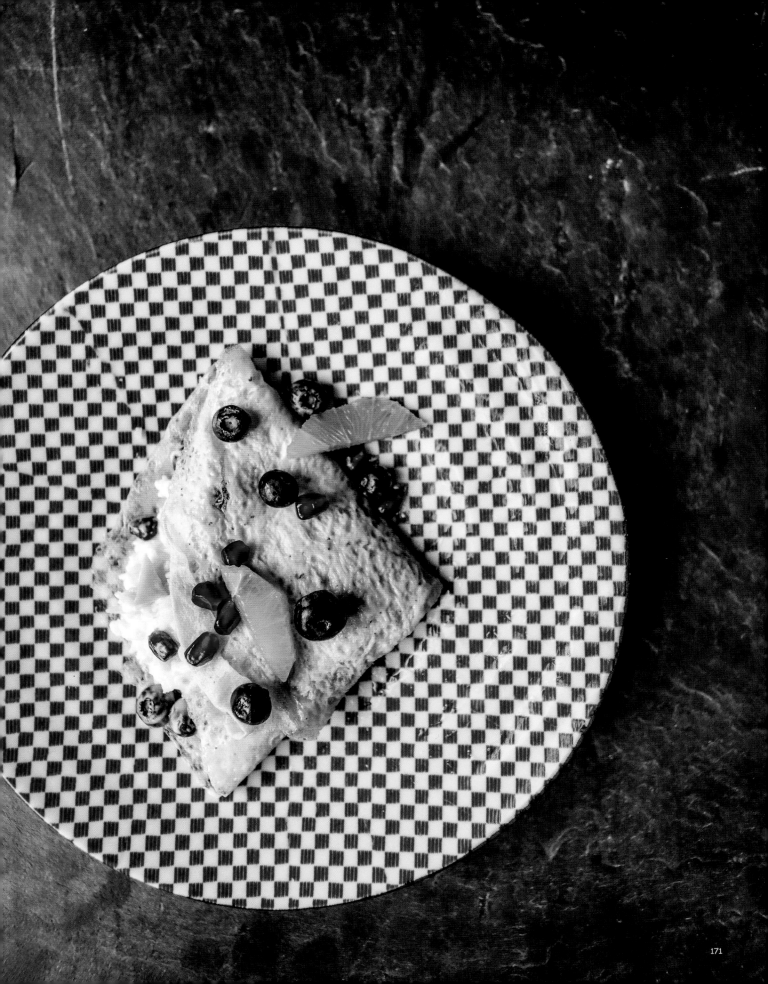

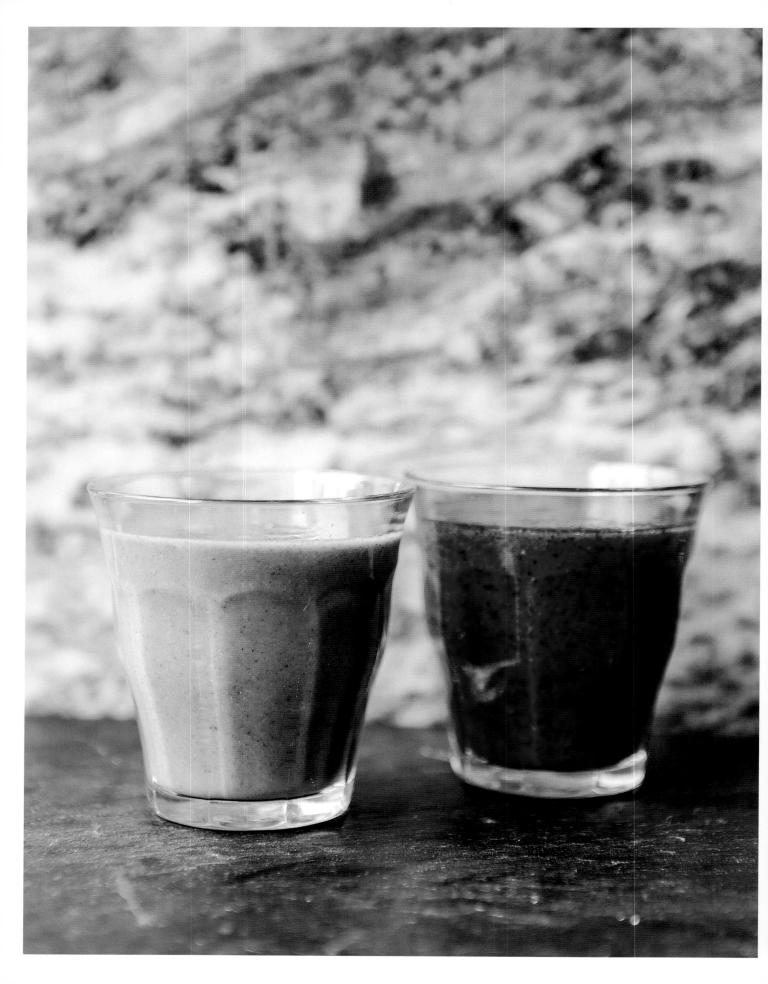

Green Goddess Smoothie

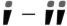

In the jug of a powerful blender, combine the greens — the spinach, kale, mint and parsley — with the kiwis, avocado, ½ of the water and ginger. Gradually purée the mixture, adding water if needed to reach the desired consistency. Season with the lime juice, honey and more of the mint leaves to taste, then serve.

TIP: Add 2 scoops of natural protein powder to turn this into a terrific recovery drink.

100 g fresh spinach, rinsed and dried

50 g fresh kale, rinsed and dried

1 handful fresh mint leaves, rinsed and dried + more to taste

1 handful fresh flat-leaf parsley leaves, rinsed and dried

2 kiwis, halved and skin removed

1 medium avocado, halved and pitted

100 mL water, divided

25 g fresh ginger, peeled and thinly sliced

Juice of 1–2 limes

Honey, to taste

Blueberry and Pineapple Protein Smoothie

In the jug of a powerful blender, combine the almond milk, blueberries, pineapple and ginger. Gradually purée the mixture, adding water if needed to reach the desired consistency. Add the protein powder and blend until well combined. Season with the lime juice and honey to taste, then serve.

300 mL almond milk

100 g frozen blueberries

100 g frozen pineapple

20 g ginger pulp or minced ginger

Zest and juice of 1 orange

40 g natural protein powder (e.g. rice, pea, whey)

Freshly squeezed lime juice, to taste

Honey, to taste

Rice and Omelet: The Time Trial Meal

In a large pot over medium-high heat, combine the water and rice, then bring them to a boil covered. Reduce the heat to medium-low, and simmer for 10-12 minutes covered. Remove the pot from the heat and set it aside for 12 minutes. Heat up a pan with 1 tbsp. of olive oil. Sauté the spinach until fully cooked, then add it to the cooked rice and combine.

Whisk the eggs together, then season with salt and pepper. In a large non-stick pan over medium-high heat, heat up the remaining olive oil. When the pan is very hot, pour ½ of the eggs into the pan. Turn the pan until the eggs are thinly spread, then cook until the they are set. Add the Parmesan and start folding the omelet from one side to the other using a heatproof rubber or silicone spatula. As you fold, move the cooked portions as far away from the heat as possible and let the parts that are still semi-liquid run to the empty part of the pan to set in a thin layer. Keep folding and making as many layers as possible so that the omelet stays velvety and fluffy. Transfer the cooked omelet from the pan onto a plate. Repeat this process with the remaining eggs. Serve the rice and spinach with the omelet and ham on the side, topped with more Parmesan and olive oil to taste.

400 mL water

200 g basmati rice, cooked

100 g baby spinach

6 whole large eggs

2 tbsp. olive oil, divided + more to taste

Salt and pepper, to taste

Freshly grated Parmesan cheese, to cook and serve

2 slices cooked ham

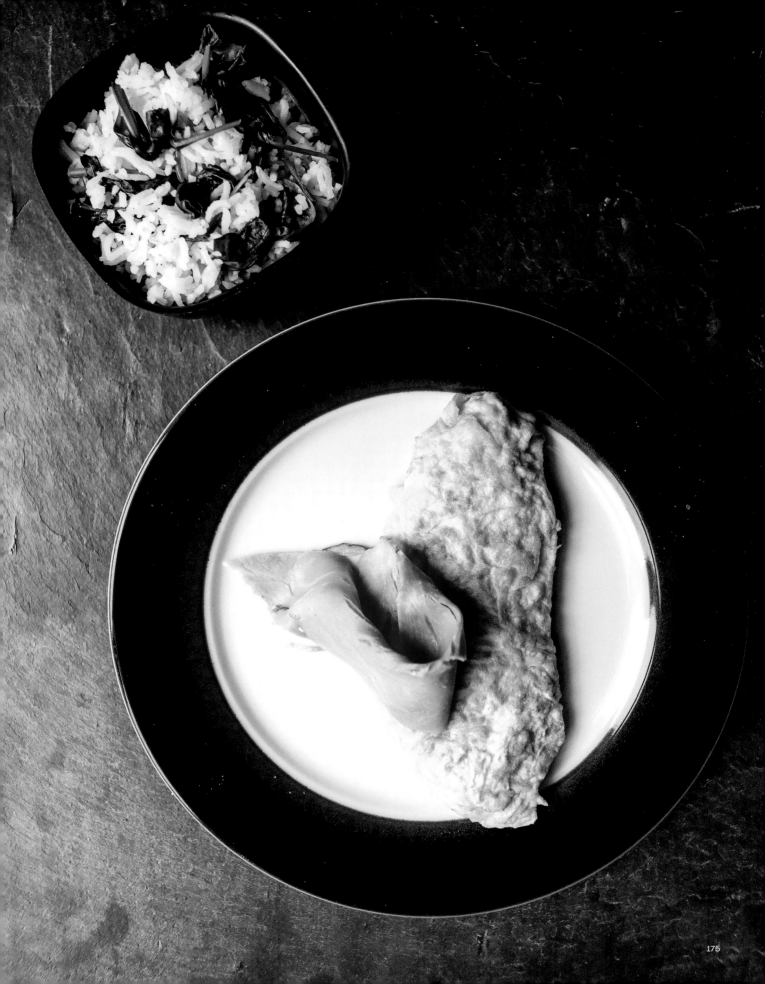

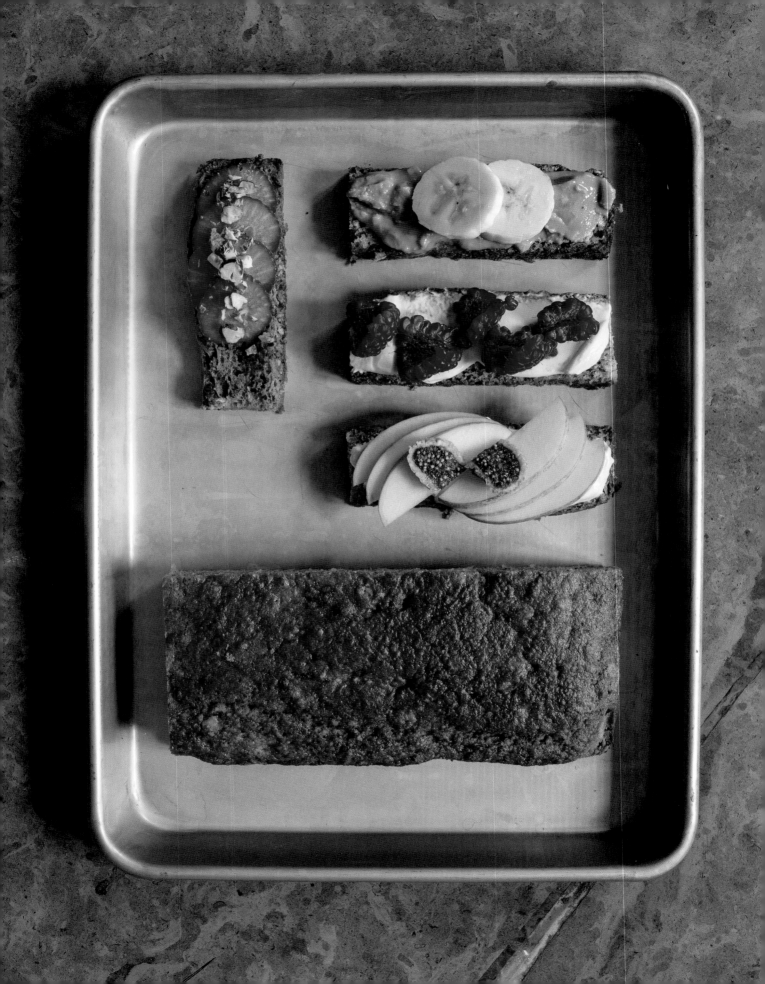

Breakfast Banana Bread

R G D V

 10

Preheat the oven to 175°C/350°F. Grease a loaf pan and line it with parchment paper. Peel and mash the bananas in a large mixing bowl and mix in the milk, sugars, olive oil and egg until well combined. Sift the flour, baking powder, salt and cardamom into the bowl containing the banana mixture using a strainer or sift. Add the almond flour and oats, then stir everything until well combined.

Transfer the mixture into the prepared pan and bake for about 40 minutes until golden and crisp on top. Remove the pan from the oven and set it aside on a wire rack to cool completely before serving.

TIP: For variations, serve with nut butter, plain Greek yogurt, and/or fresh berries.

3 ripe, brown bananas

200 mL non-dairy milk

100 g brown sugar

50 g brown cane sugar

45 mL olive oil

1 whole large egg

200 g flour

3 tsp. baking powder

½ tsp. salt

½ tsp. ground cardamom

140 g almond flour

115 g oats

Coconut-rice Pancakes with Vanilla Yogurt and Lime

(Re) (G) (V)

In a large mixing bowl, combine the rice, eggs, banana, coconut flour, cinnamon and salt. Stir until well combined. In a large non-stick pan over medium heat, heat up the olive oil. Add 3 small spoons of the batter and cook for 4 minutes on each side until golden. Transfer the pancakes onto a plate and cover with tin foil to keep warm. Repeat this process until all of the batter is used.

—

In a small mixing bowl, combine the yogurt and the vanilla seeds. Stir until well combined, then season with lime zest, juice and honey to taste. Serve the pancakes with the yogurt mixture and fruits topped with shaved coconut.

250 g cooked rice

2 whole large eggs

1 banana, mashed

50 g coconut flour

¼ tsp. ground cinnamon

1 pinch salt

1 tsp. olive oil

200 g plain Greek yogurt

1 vanilla bean

Zest and juice of 2 limes

Honey, to taste

Fresh assorted fruit, to serve

Toasted shaved coconut, to serve

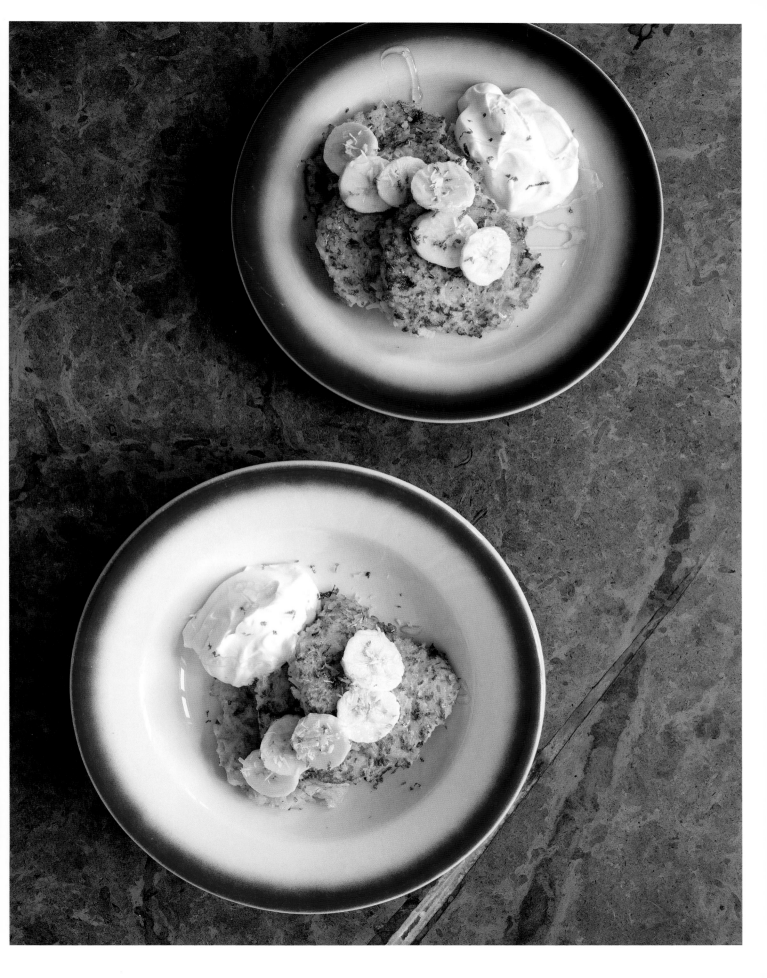

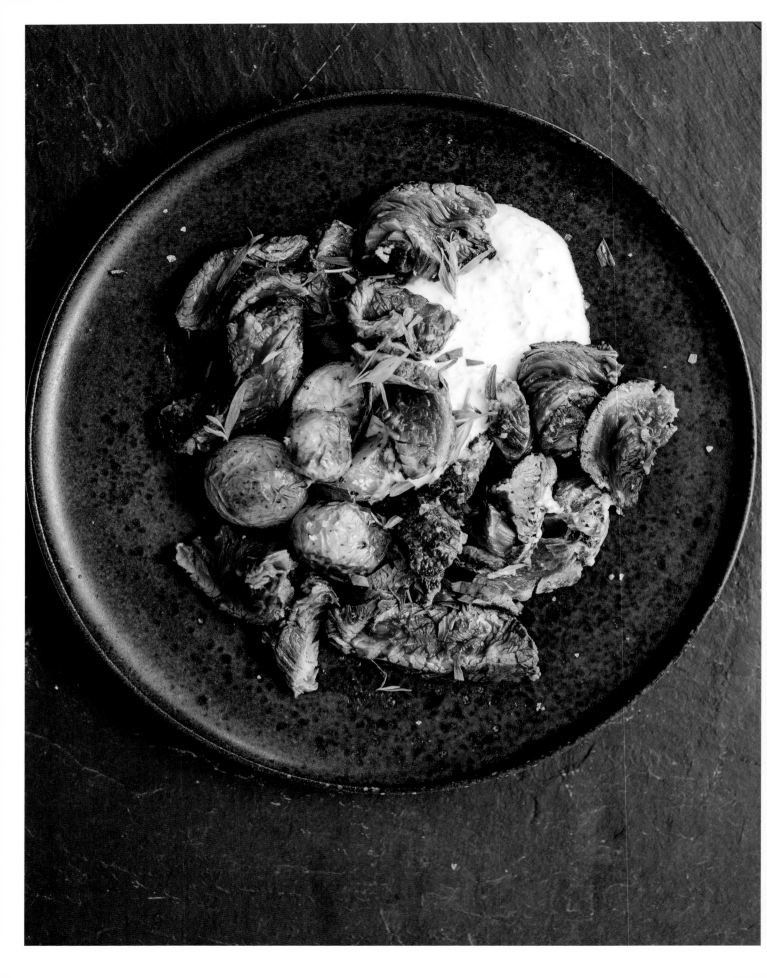

Onglet de Boeuf 'Béarnaise'

Preheat the oven to 200°C/390°F. Line a baking sheet with parchment paper. Scrub and wash the potatoes; halving them if necessary. Cut the garlic heads across the bulbs and toss them all with the olive oil, rosemary, salt and pepper. Spread them out evenly onto the prepared sheet, then roast in the oven for 20-25 minutes until golden brown and tender.

———

Peel and mince the shallot and marinate it in the apple cider vinegar. Rinse, pick and chop the tarragon. Combine the shallot, tarragon, yogurt and mustard in a bowl, then season with salt and pepper.

———

Season the beef with salt and pepper and heat up a frying pan with 2 tbsp. of oil. Cook the beef for 2-3 minutes on each side until the red juices come through. Remove it from the pan and set it aside to rest for at least 5 minutes before serving. Slice the beef thinly, then season with flaky salt and pepper. Serve with the potatoes and cold yogurt 'Béarnaise'.

1000 g new potatoes

2 whole heads garlic

60 mL olive oil, divided

2 sprigs fresh rosemary, picked

1 large banana shallot

3 tbsp. apple cider vinegar

½ bunch fresh tarragon

200 g plain Greek yogurt

1 tbsp. Dijon mustard

600 g onglet or hanger steak

200 g plain Greek yogurt

Flaky salt and pepper, to serve

Beef Tartar with Egg Yolk and Bitter Salad

1 bunch fresh flat-leaf parsley

1 bunch fresh tarragon

2 medium shallots

1 head radicchio or bitter salad

300 g lean beef (tell your butcher it is for a tartar)

2 tbsp. whole grain mustard

2 tbsp. olive oil

2 eggs

Salt and pepper, to taste

4 slices of bread, to serve

G D N

Rinse, pick and finely chop the parsley and tarragon. Peel and mince the shallots. Rinse and tear the salad. Wash your cutting board, and put on disposable gloves. Finely dice or mince the beef, then combine it with the fresh herbs, shallots, mustard and olive oil. Season with salt and pepper.

—

Wash your hands and carefully crack the eggs into a bowl. With your clean fingers, lift the egg yolks out and carefully pinch the white strings with your index and middle fingers. Arrange a small portion of tartar on a plate and make a space in the middle to place the yolk. Grill or toast the bread and serve with the tartar.

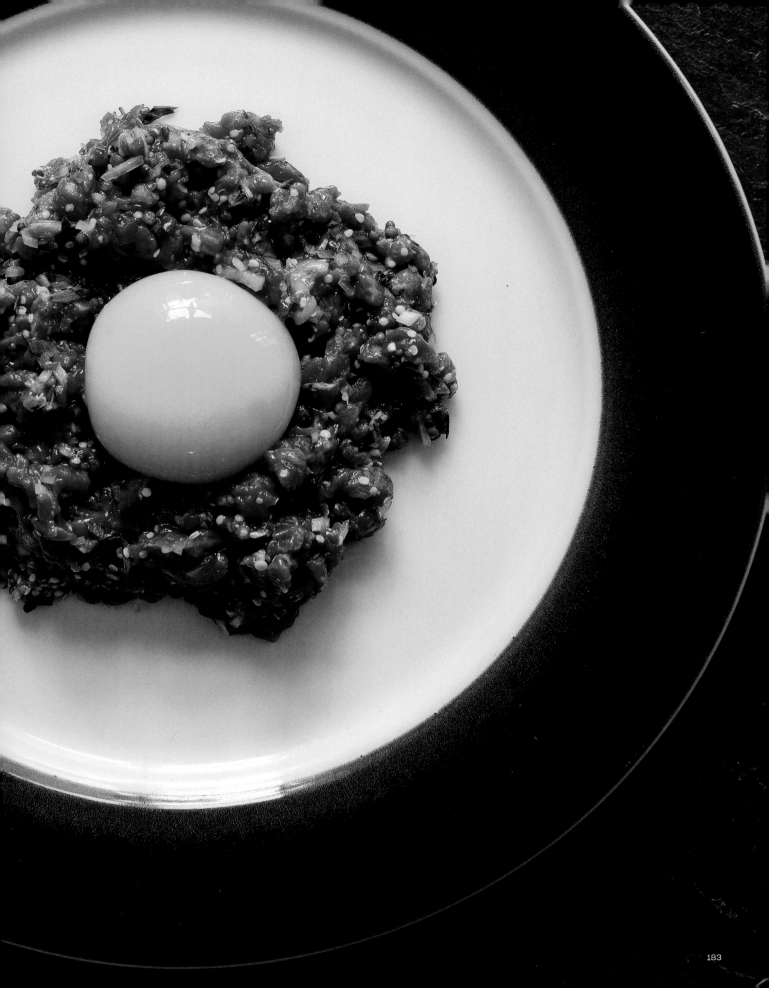

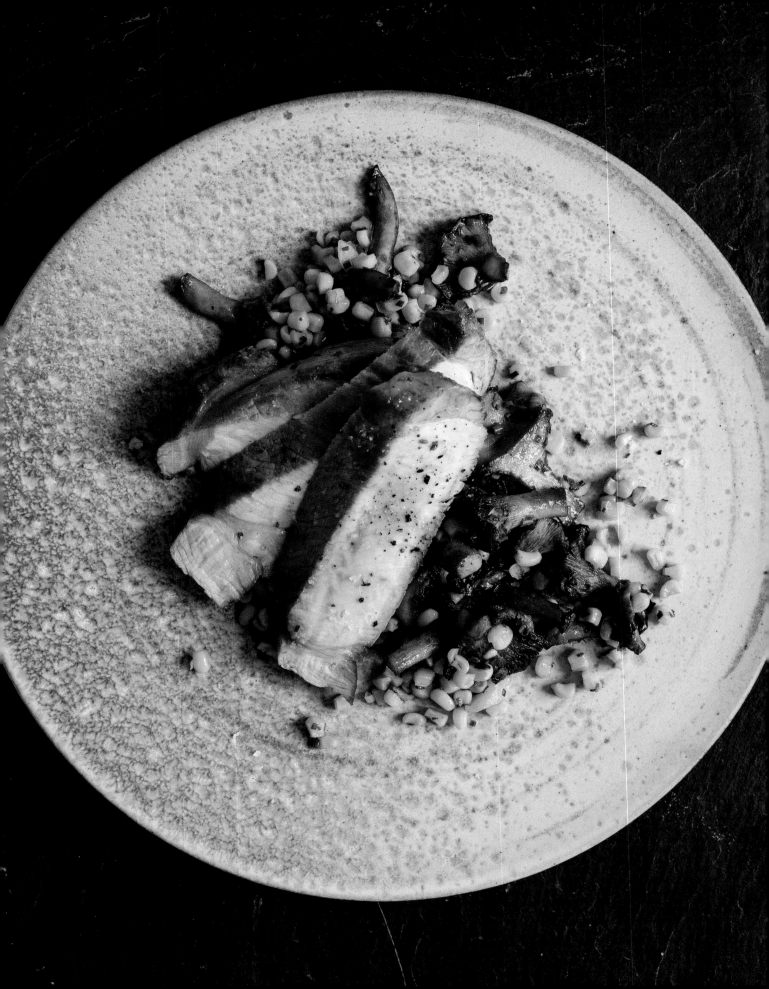

Organic Pork Chops, Fresh Corn, and Chanterelles

Carefully rinse the mushrooms, cut off the roots, and let them air-dry on a piece of paper towel. Remove the husks and cut the corn off the cobs, then discard the cobs. Peel and slice the garlic thinly. Rinse and pick the thyme. Mince the chives.

In a large frying pan over medium heat, warm 2 tbsp. of olive oil. Fry the mushrooms until golden brown without stirring too much since they will release water and start boiling. Add the thyme, then season with salt and pepper to taste. Remove the mushrooms from the pan and wipe it clean. Heat up the pan again and sauté the corn for about 2-3 minutes until sweet and fully cooked. Add the mushrooms and chives, then season with salt and pepper to taste.

Season the pork chops with salt and pepper, then heat up the pan over medium-high heat with 1 tbsp. of oil. Fry the pork chops for 3-4 minutes on each side, depending on their thickness.
Remove them from the heat and set them aside to rest for at least 5 minutes. Slice the meat, then season with salt and pepper.
Plate them on top of the mushrooms and corn garnish, then serve with soft polenta.

250 g chanterelle mushrooms

2 cobs corn

2 cloves garlic

½ bunch fresh thyme

1 bunch fresh chives

600 g organic pork chops on the bone

4 tbsp. olive oil, divided

Soft polenta for serving (see recipe on p.186)

Soft Polenta

Bring the water to a boil, add the salt, and lower the heat. Whisk in the polenta as it comes to a boil again. Cook while whisking for 5 minutes until the polenta is smooth and soft. Add water if needed until it reaches a desired consistency, then add the Parmesan and season with salt, pepper, lemon zest and juice to taste.

———

TIP: For variations, try the suggestions below –
· Add pine seeds and chopped basil
· Add a blend of mixed fresh herbs
· Substitute Parmesan for mascarpone

800 mL water

1 tsp. salt

200 g fine polenta

100 g shredded Parmesan cheese

Zest and juice of 1 lemon

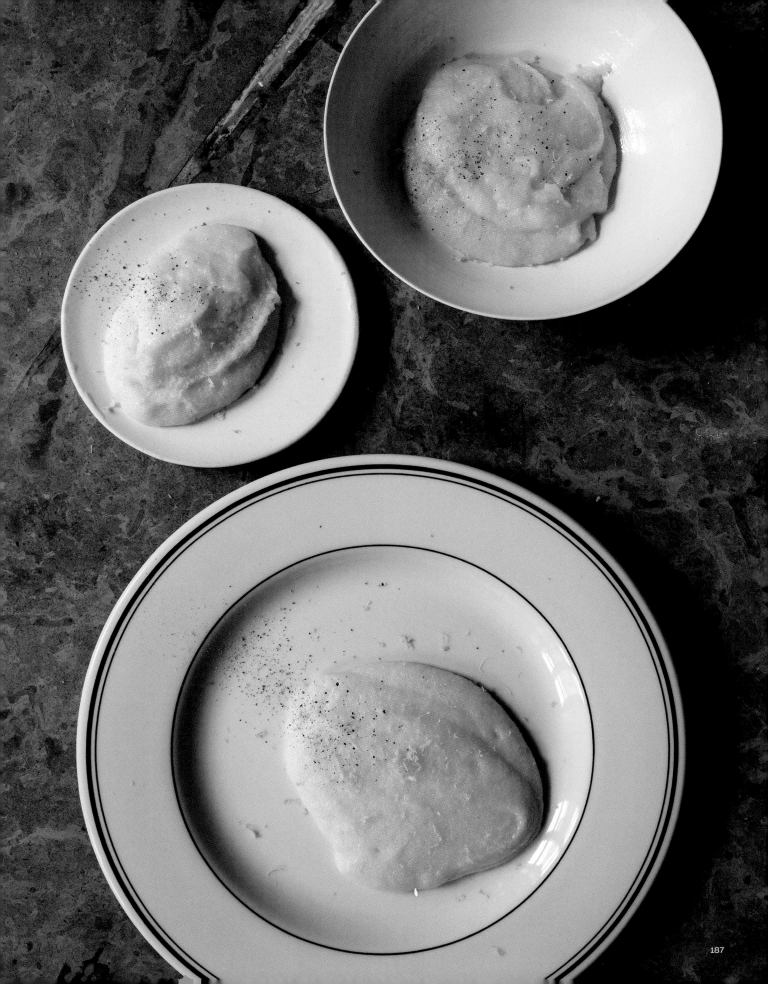

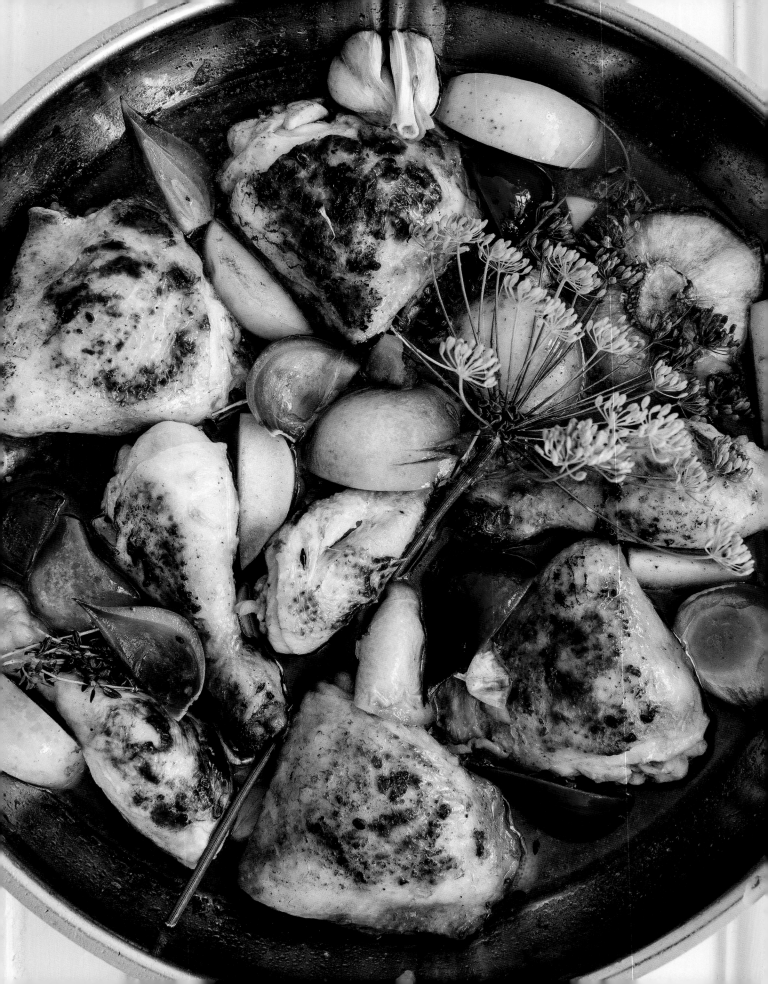

1-pot Chicken
with Apple, Onion, and Crown Dill

Rinse the apples and lemons. Quarter the apples and cut out the cores. Peel the onions and quarter them. Halve the garlic heads horizontally across all the bulbs. Divide the chicken legs in half by cutting through the joints with a sharp knife. To locate the correct spot to cut, move the leg back and forth while searching with your fingers for the little gap by the tip of the joint. Season the chicken with salt and pepper.

In a large sauté pan or Dutch oven, heat up the olive oil and brown the skin of the chicken. Add the apples, onions, garlic, thyme and dill to the pan, then pour the apple juice and apple cider vinegar over the mixture. Bring them to a boil and reduce the heat to low, then cook covered for 30–35 minutes until the chicken is tender and the onions are fully cooked. Remove them from the pan and set them aside on a plate covered with tin foil.

Return the pan to the heat and cook until the sauce's volume reduces down by half. Stir in the butter. Season with salt, pepper and vinegar to taste. Place the chicken back onto the pan and garnish with the fresh chervil. Serve with the crushed potatoes.

3 medium apples

3 lemons

3 red onions

2 whole garlic heads

4 whole chicken legs

2 tbsp. olive oil

1 handful lemon thyme

2 crowns dill or fennel flower

200 mL apple juice

100 mL apple cider vinegar + more to taste

20 g butter (optional)

Salt and pepper, to taste

1 bunch fresh chervil, rinsed

Crushed potatoes, to serve (see recipe on p.190)

Crushed New Potatoes with Herbs

G D N V

Scrub the potatoes clean, leave the skin on, and bring them to a boil in unsalted water. Turn down the heat to medium and cook for about 15 minutes until the potatoes are a little overcooked.

—

Rinse and pick the parsley, then chop it finely. Peel and grate the garlic. Strain the potatoes and crush them with a large whisk. Add the olive oil, parsley, garlic and lemon zest. Season with salt, pepper and lemon juice to taste. Serve immediately or plate it in an ovenproof dish, sprinkle some Parmesan, then bake it just before serving until hot and golden.

1 kg new potatoes
½ bunch parsley
Zest and juice of 2 lemons
1 bulb garlic
Olive oil, to cook
Salt and pepper, to taste
Freshly grated Parmesan cheese, to serve

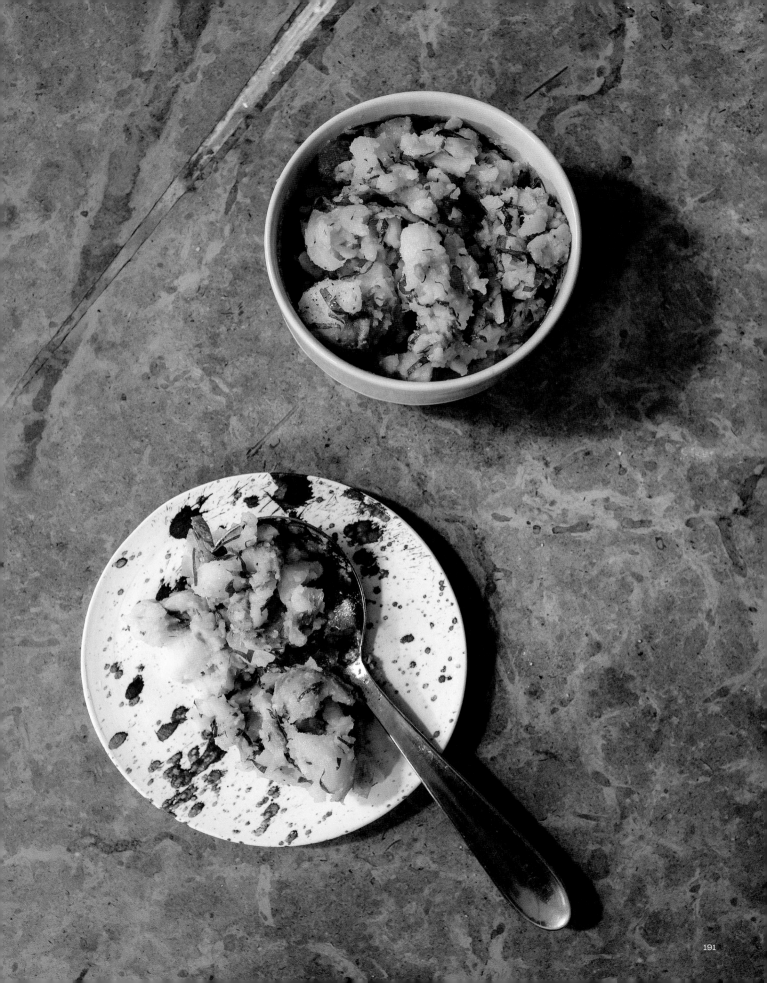

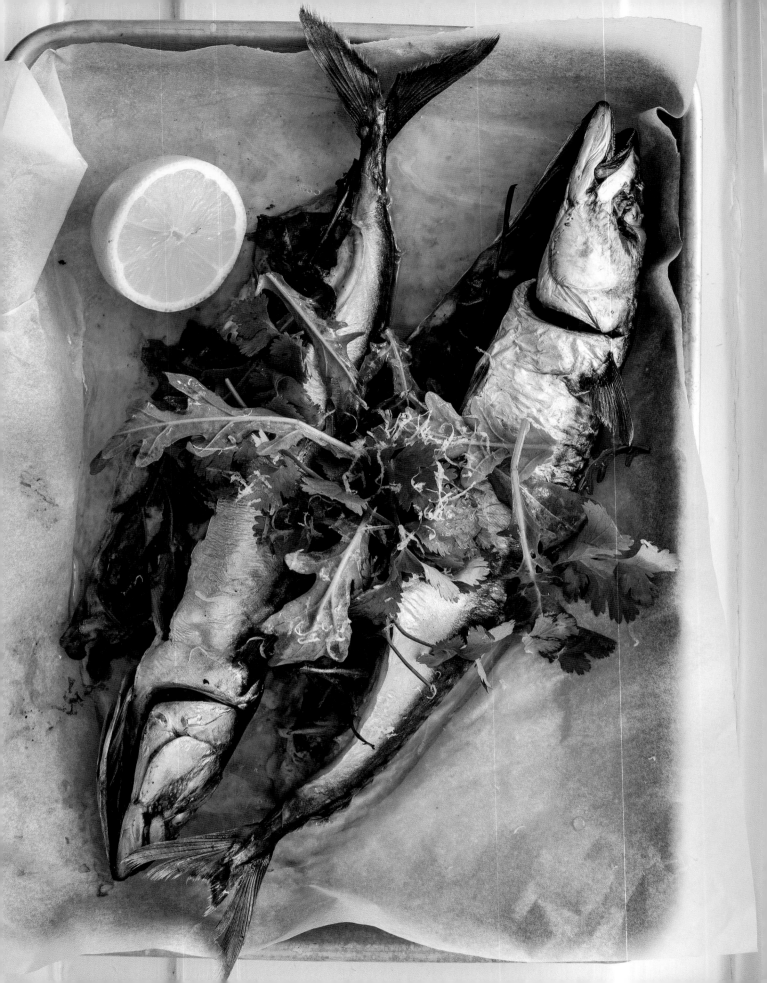

Whole Stuffed Mackerel
with Arugula, Fresh Coriander, and Lemon

Preheat the oven to 200°C/390°F. Line a baking sheet with parchment paper. Gut the mackerels and rinse them well (you can also ask your fishmonger to gut and debone them for you, in which case you can just rinse them).

Using a sharp knife, make an incision on the inside of the fish from the belly all the way to the tail. Using your index fingers, push through the flesh underneath the spine and just underneath the head. With your thumb holding onto the top of the spine, crack it. Place your middle and index fingers of 1 hand on each side of the spine. Carefully wiggle your fingers along it to loosen the flesh from the bone, without pulling off too much flesh. Using your other hand, push the flesh down from the rib bones and pull the spine loose. Once the spine has been completely removed, crack off the tail and discard it. Check for any leftover bones; if you find any, discard them. Place the deboned fish on the prepared sheet, then season with salt and pepper. Repeat this process with the remaining fish.

Wash your hands and the cutting board well. Rinse the arugula and coriander. Pick the coriander, then peel and slice the garlic. Divide the arugula and coriander into 2 bowls, then combine the garlic, olive oil and the zest and juice of 1 lemon in one. Season with salt and pepper.

Stuff the mackerels with the mixture and bake for about 8-10 minutes until a cake tester slides through the flesh with no resistance. (Check periodically during the cooking time to ensure that they do not overcook.) Toss the remaining arugula and coriander with olive oil, lemon zest and juice. Season with salt and pepper. Serve the baked mackerels topped with arugula, coriander and roasted potatoes on the side.

4 small whole mackerels

250 g fresh arugula

1 bunch fresh coriander

4 cloves garlic

Zest and juice of 2 lemons

60 mL olive oil + more as needed

Salt and pepper, to taste

Roasted potatoes, to serve

Vegetable and Halloumi Skewers with Tahini Sauce

G D N V

Preheat the oven to 200°C/395°F. Line a baking sheet with parchment paper or light up the grill. Rinse all the vegetables. Core the peppers and cut them into bite-sized pieces. Peel the onions and cut them into wedges. Dice the squash and halloumi.

Soak 16 wooden skewers in water. Skewer the vegetables, halloumi cheese and tomatoes. Drizzle them with olive oil, then season with salt and pepper to taste. Grill or roast for about 15-20 minutes until the vegetables are tender and roasted.

In a small mixing bowl, combine the honey, tahini, garlic, lemon zest and juice. Season with salt and pepper to taste, then stir until well combined. Adjust the consistency by adding water if needed. Serve the skewers with grilled meat/fish or with steamed rice/quinoa.

2 medium red peppers

2 medium red onions

1 zucchini squash

200 g halloumi cheese

100 g cherry tomatoes

Olive oil, for drizzling

2 tbsp. honey

4 tbsp. tahini

1 clove garlic, minced

Zest and juice of 1 lemon

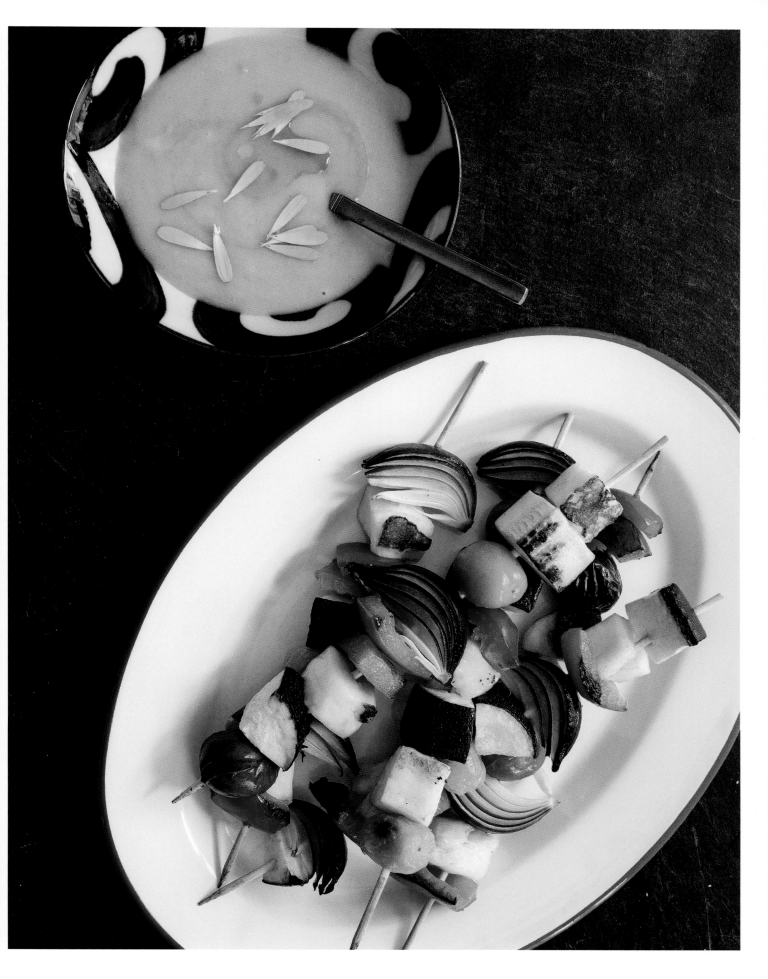

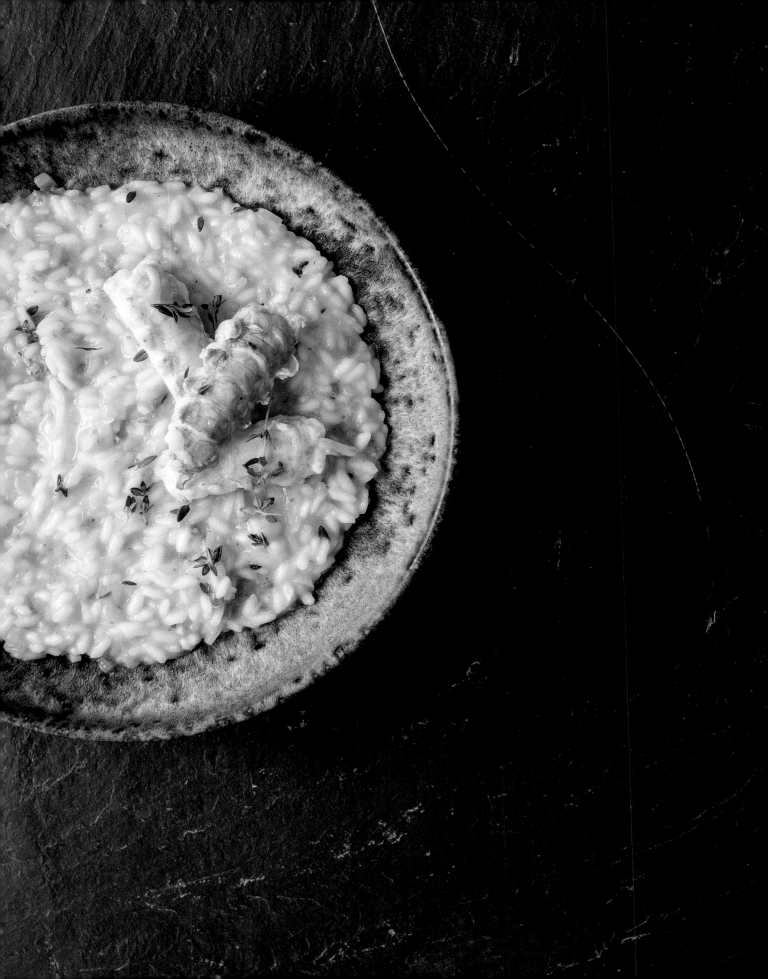

Risotto with Langoustines and Lemon Thyme

Peel the langoustines by gently pulling off their heads. Press the 2 long sides of the tails together to crack the back. Gently pull the shell apart to release the tail. Pinch the middle tail blade as you pull off the shell to remove the intestines. With a sharp knife, halve the langoustine heads. Scoop the tomalley (soft green substance) out, chop it, and put it aside for later. In a sauté pan, fry the langoustine heads in 2 tbsp. of olive oil until they are bright red. Add ½ of the bunch of thyme as well as the wine and 200 mL of water. Bring them to a boil, then reduce the heat to simmer for 5 minutes. Strain the broth and discard the shells and thyme.

—

Peel and mince the garlic and shallots. In a large pot or sauté pan, sauté them with 2 tbsp. of olive oil over medium heat until tender. Add the tomalley and sauté until bright red. Add the rice and sauté for 2 minutes until everything is well combined. Pour the stock over the rice and simmer for about 2 minutes until it has reduced to ⅓ of the volume. Add ⅓ of the water and cook; stirring constantly with a wooden spoon until the rice has absorbed all the liquid. Repeat this process with the remaining water until the rice is tender with a bite. Finish the risotto off by leaving a little excess liquid for serving, since it will set while the langoustines are cooking. Add the Parmesan and 100mL of oil, then stir until the mixture is creamy. Season the risotto with salt, pepper, lemon zest and juice to taste. Remove it from the heat.

—

Heat up a frying pan with 2 tbsp. of olive oil. Sprinkle the pan with a pinch of salt and place the langoustine tails with their backs down. Fry for about 30 seconds, flip them over, and remove the pan from the heat. Serve the risotto in a deep plate and top with the fried tails and the thyme.

8 large fresh whole langoustines

1 bunch fresh lemon thyme

2 cloves garlic

2 medium shallots

500 g risotto rice

300 mL white wine

1200 mL water

200 g freshly grated Parmesan cheese

100 mL olive oil

Zest and juice of 2 lemons

Salt and pepper, to taste

Cold Pea Soup with Parsley and Mint

G D N V

Peel and mince the shallots and garlic. Rinse and pick the herbs separately. Mince ½ of the mint finely and save it for serving. In a large pot over medium heat, warm the 1 tbsp. of olive oil. Add the shallots and garlic, then sauté for 2 minutes until tender. Add the white wine, bring it to a boil over medium heat, and reduce it down by ⅓. Add the stock and bring it to a boil. Add the frozen peas, parsley and the mint not minced into the soup, then allow it to reach a low simmer. Transfer the broth into a clean container and let it cool down in an ice bath or in the refrigerator until it is about room temperature.

Blend the soup until completely smooth. Add 50 mL of olive oil and season with salt, pepper, lime zest and juice to taste. Blend it again and let the soup cool down completely. Serve it in bowls topped with fresh peas and the minced mint.

TIP: To make the soup into a main course, serve it warm with baked fish and bread.

2 medium shallots

1 clove garlic

½ bunch fresh flat-leaf parsley

½ bunch fresh mint

50 mL +1 tbsp. cold-pressed olive oil, divided

200 mL white wine

1000 mL vegetable stock or water

400 g frozen peas

Zest and juice of 2 limes

Salt and pepper, to taste

100 g fresh shelled peas

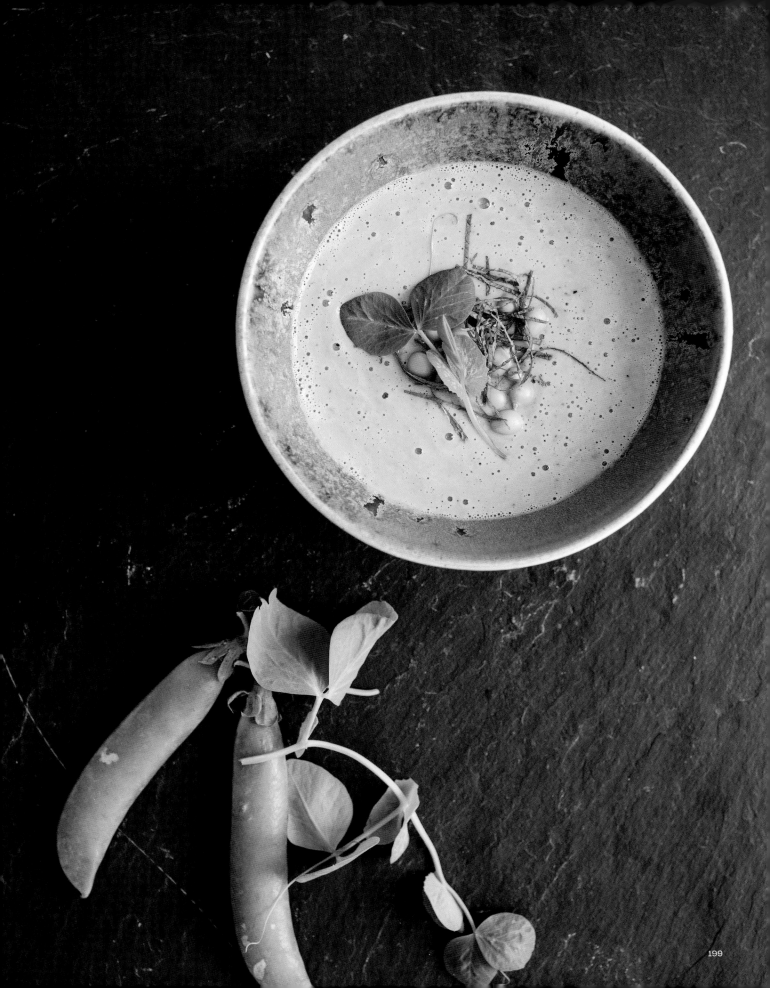

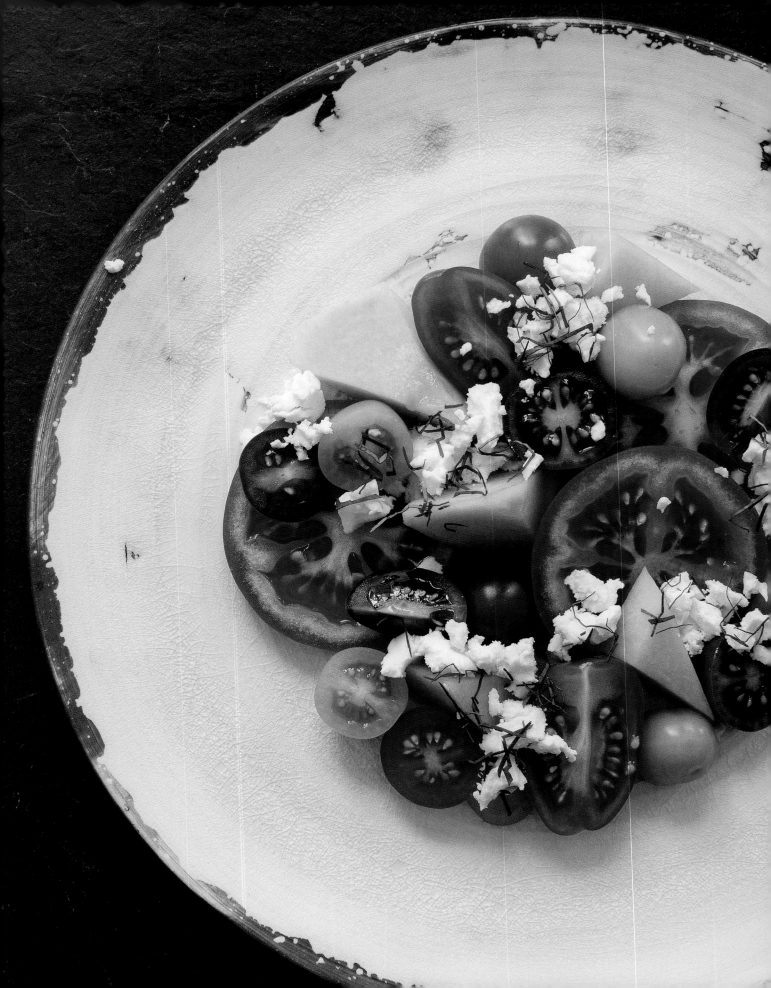

Tomato-melon Salad with Feta Cheese

Rinse all the tomatoes. Halve the small ones and slice the large ones, then season with salt and pepper. Halve the melon and scrape out the seeds. Cut off the rinds and dice the flesh into bite-sized pieces. Rinse, pick and mince the coriander finely.
Arrange the tomatoes and melon on a large serving platter, then top them with crumbled cheese and the minced coriander to serve.

500 g small ripe tomatoes

2 large ripe tomatoes

1 medium cantaloupe

100 g feta or goat cheese

½ bunch fresh coriander or cilantro, minced

Olive oil, for drizzling

Salt and pepper, to taste

Lentil Salad with Grilled Eggplant, Pesto, and Strawberries

Peel the carrots, onion and garlic. Quarter the onion and cut the carrots into large chunks. Rinse and pick the parsley, then tie the stems together with twine. In a large pot, cover the lentils with stock. Add 1 tsp. of salt, the carrots, onion, 3 cloves of garlic and parsley stems. Bring them to a boil and reduce the heat to medium-low. Cover and cook for 20-30 minutes until the lentils are tender but still with texture (they should not be mushy). Strain the lentils and discard the carrots, onion and stems.

Blend the basil, olive oil, ½ of the parsley and ½ of the lemon zest until semi-smooth. Add the pine seeds and Parmesan in small chunks, then blend until the pesto reaches the desired consistency. Season with salt, pepper and lemon juice to taste.

Slice the eggplants into 1 cm-thick slices, lightly salt them on both sides, and let them sit for 5 minutes. Dab them with a paper towel, then grill or fry them with olive oil on a pan over high heat until dark brown and tender.

Rinse the strawberries and slice or quarter them. Combine the lentils, eggplant, strawberries and the rest of the parsley with ½ of the pesto. Season with salt, pepper and lemon juice to taste. Serve in a large serving bowl topped with some fresh strawberries, parsley and the remaining pesto on the side.

2 carrots

1 onion

4 cloves garlic

1 bunch fresh flat-leaf parsley

300 g green or Puy lentils

1000 mL water or stock

1 bunch fresh basil

200 mL olive oil + more to fry

50 g pine seeds

100 g Parmesan cheese

Zest and juice of 2 lemons

1 large eggplant

100 g fresh strawberries

Salt and pepper, to taste

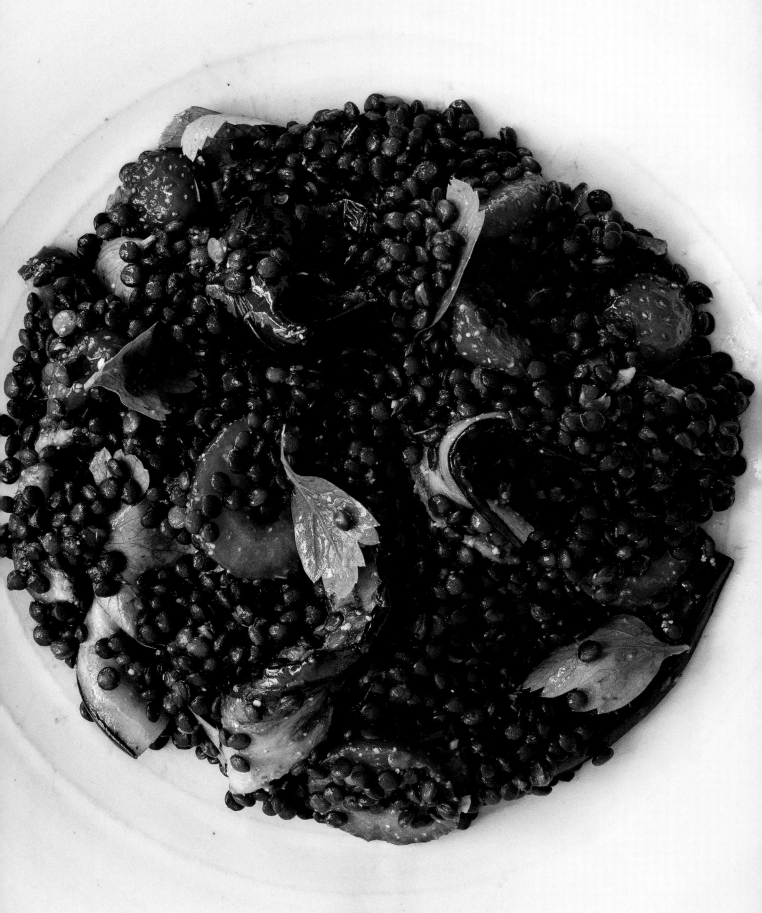

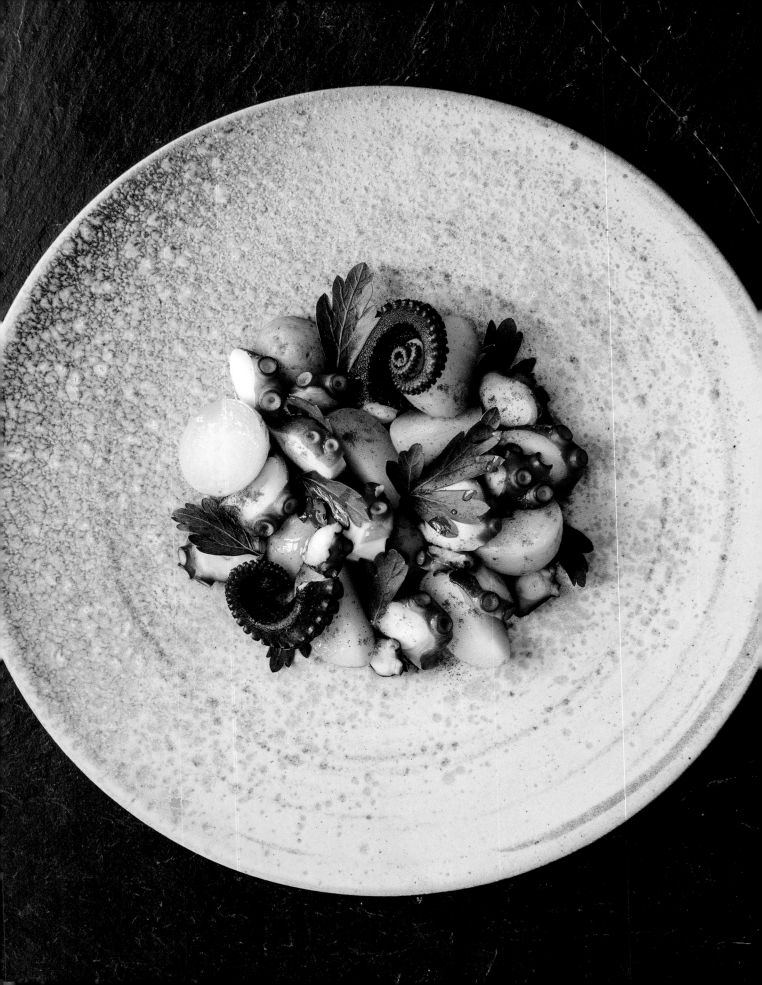

Octopus a la Gallega

Rinse and clean the octopus thoroughly under cold running water. In a large stockpot over medium heat, bring the salted water, wine, cinnamon stick and the bay leaves to a boil. Slowly dip the octopus, tentacles first, into the boiling liquid until the tentacles curl up nicely. Submerge the whole octopus until it returns to a boil. Reduce the heat to low and simmer for 45 minutes. Check to see if the octopus is tender by piercing a cake tester through one of the thick tentacles. Remove the pot from the heat and set it aside to rest for 30 minutes. Discard the liquid and cut the octopus into ½ cm-thick pieces.

———

In a large pot, cover the potatoes with the lightly salted water, and bring them to a boil over medium heat. Reduce the heat to medium and cook for 10 minutes. Remove the pot from the heat and set it aside to rest for 5–7 minutes. Drain the water. Halve the larger potatoes, then season them with salt, pepper, oil, lemon zest and juice. Rinse and pick the parsley. To serve, plate the potatoes, octopus and parsley, then sprinkle with the smoked paprika.

1 octopus (1 kg)

2 L salted water

500 mL red wine

1 stick cinnamon

4 bay leaves

500 g new potatoes

Lightly salted water, to cover

Zest and juice of 1 lemon

2 tbsp. olive oil

1 handful fresh flat-leaf parsley

½ tsp. smoked paprika

Salt and pepper, to taste

Salmorejo (Cold Tomato Soup)

Dice the tomatoes. Peel the onion and garlic, then quarter them. Cut the bread into chunks. Place the tomatoes, onion, garlic, and bread in a heat-proof bowl, then pour the boiling water over it. Ensure that everything is covered, and set the bowl aside for 1 hour. Strain 300 mL of the liquid and set it aside. Discard the rest of the liquid, and squeeze any excess out of the bread.

Blend the soaked ingredients to a smooth consistency, adding from the 300 mL of liquid if needed to adjust texture. While the blender is running, add the olive oil, then season with the sherry vinegar, salt and pepper to taste. Let the soup cool down completely. Bring a casserole of salted water to a boil, submerge the eggs, and let them boil for 8 minutes. Cool the eggs down under coldrunning water. Once the eggs have chilled, peel and dice or shred them. Slice the ham into smaller pieces and mince the chives. Serve the ice-cold soup in deep plates topped with the eggs, ham, olive oil and chives.

6 very ripe tomatoes

1 small onion

1 clove garlic

4 slices day-old bread

Boiling water, to cover

100 mL olive oil

Sherry vinegar, to taste

4 whole large eggs

4 slices dried ham

1 bunch chives, sliced

Salt and pepper, to taste

Fresh bread, to serve

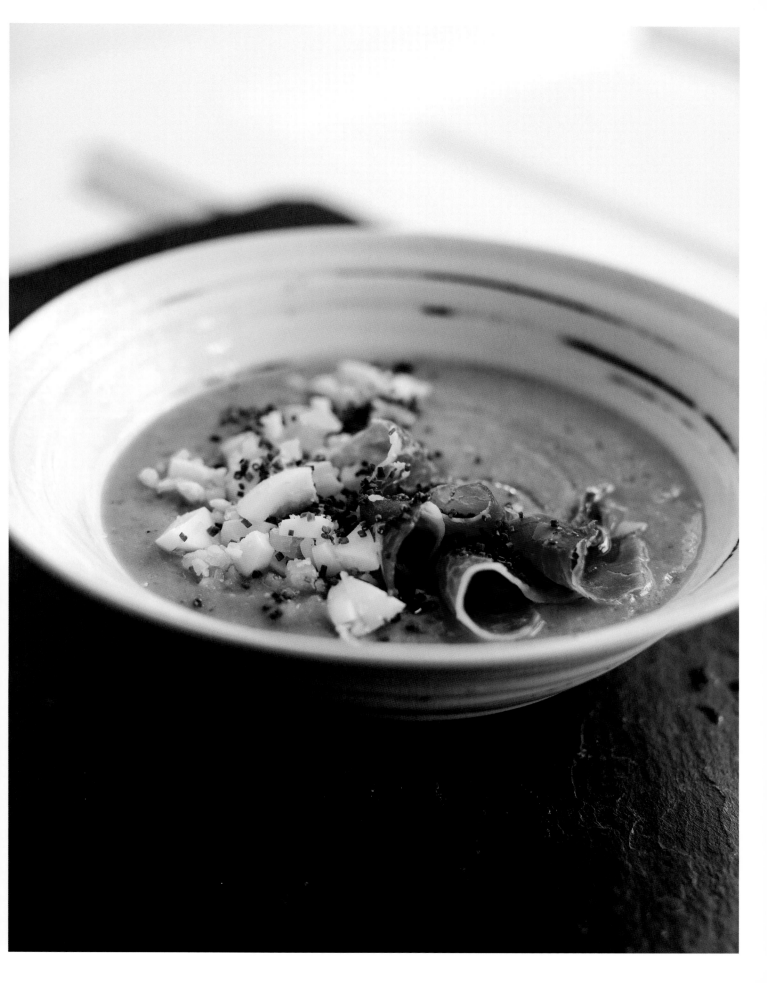

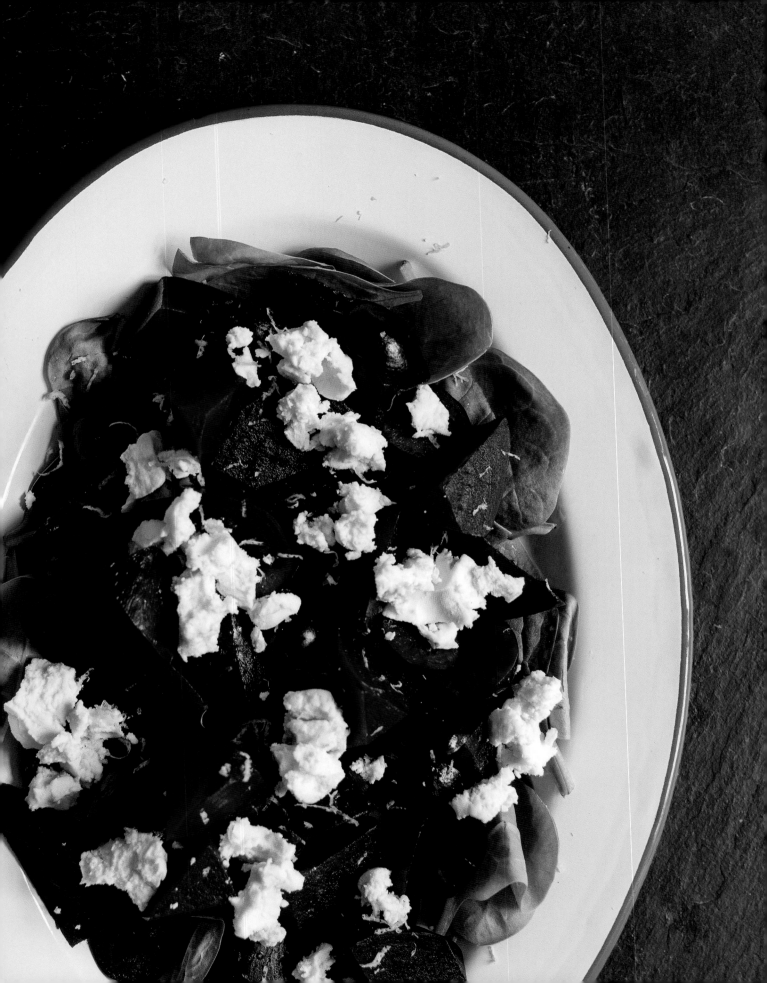

Beets and Baby Spinach with Lime and Sesame Vinaigrette

Scrub the beets and bring them to a boil in a large pot with unsalted water. Reduce the heat to medium-low and simmer for about 45 minutes until all the beets are tender. Pierce a cake tester through the beets. If it slides through easily, they are done. Put on single-use gloves and squeeze the skin off the beets. Cut them into bite-sized pieces.

Rinse and spin the spinach in a salad spinner. In a small mixing bowl, combine the lime zest and juice, lemon juice, honey and garlic. Whisk in the olive oil, then season with salt, pepper and sesame oil to taste. Marinate the beets in half of the dressing. Plate the beets and spinach on a serving platter, then sprinkle them with goat cheese and lemon zest. Serve the rest of the dressing on the side.

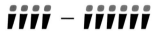

1 kg beets

1 lemon, zest and juice

250 g baby spinach

1 lime, zest and juice

1 tbsp. honey

1 clove garlic

100 mL cold-pressed olive oil

1 tbsp. toasted sesame oil

100 g goat cheese or burrata

Salt and pepper, to taste

Plums, Fennel, and Radicchio with Tarragon and Toasted Hazelnuts

Ⓖ Ⓓ Ⓥ

Preheat the oven to 175°C/345°F. Line a baking sheet with parchment paper. Rinse the plums, halve and pit them, then cut them into wedges. Rinse the fennel, trim the brown parts off, then slice it thinly on a Japanese mandolin. Submerge the sliced fennel into cold water with lemon juice. Break the radicchio into bite-sized pieces, then rinse and spin them in a salad spinner. Rinse, pick and chop the fresh tarragon.

—

Toss the hazelnuts onto the prepared sheet and toast for 10–15 minutes until golden brown. Remove the sheet from the oven and set them aside to cool completely. Once cool, roll the hazelnuts between your hands to get the shells off. Discard the shells, and chop the hazelnuts roughly.

—

In a small mixing bowl, combine the apple cider vinegar and mustard. While whisking, drizzle in the olive oil and mix in the tarragon. Season with salt, pepper and more apple cider vinegar to taste. Toss the plums, fennel and radicchio into the mixture, then serve on a large platter after sprinkling with hazelnuts. Serve the rest of the dressing on the side.

2 medium plums

2 medium bulbs fennel

Juice of 1 lemon

1 head radicchio salad

½ bunch fresh tarragon

50 g whole hazelnuts

20 mL apple cider vinegar + more to taste

20 g grainy or Dijon mustard

100 mL olive oil

Salt and pepper, to taste

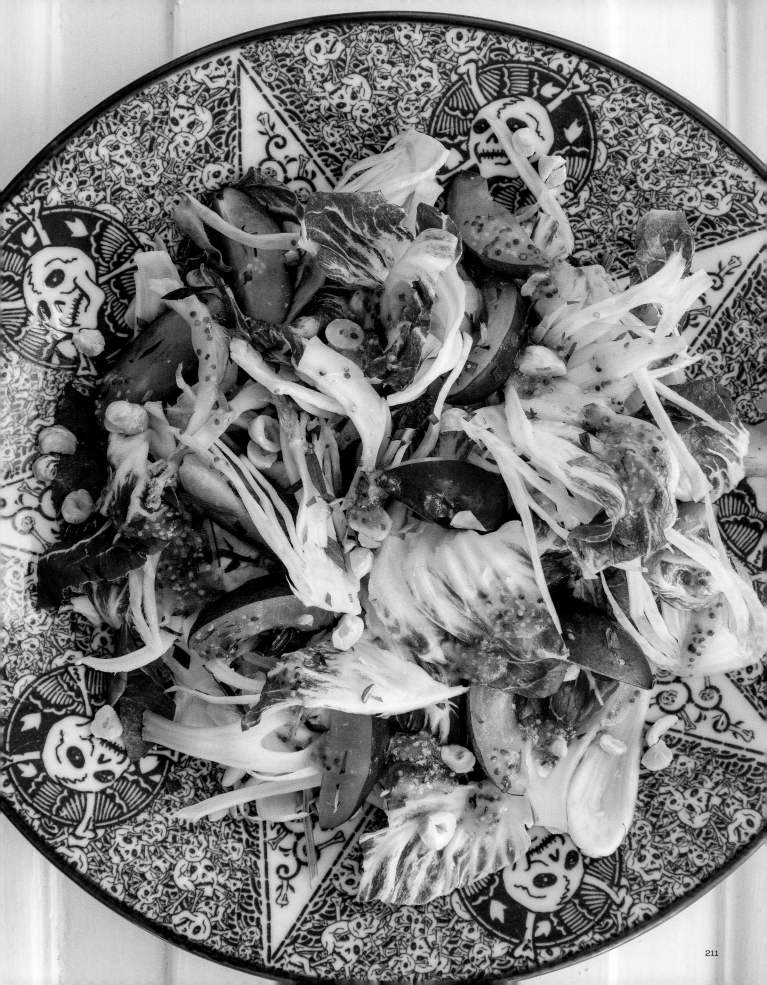

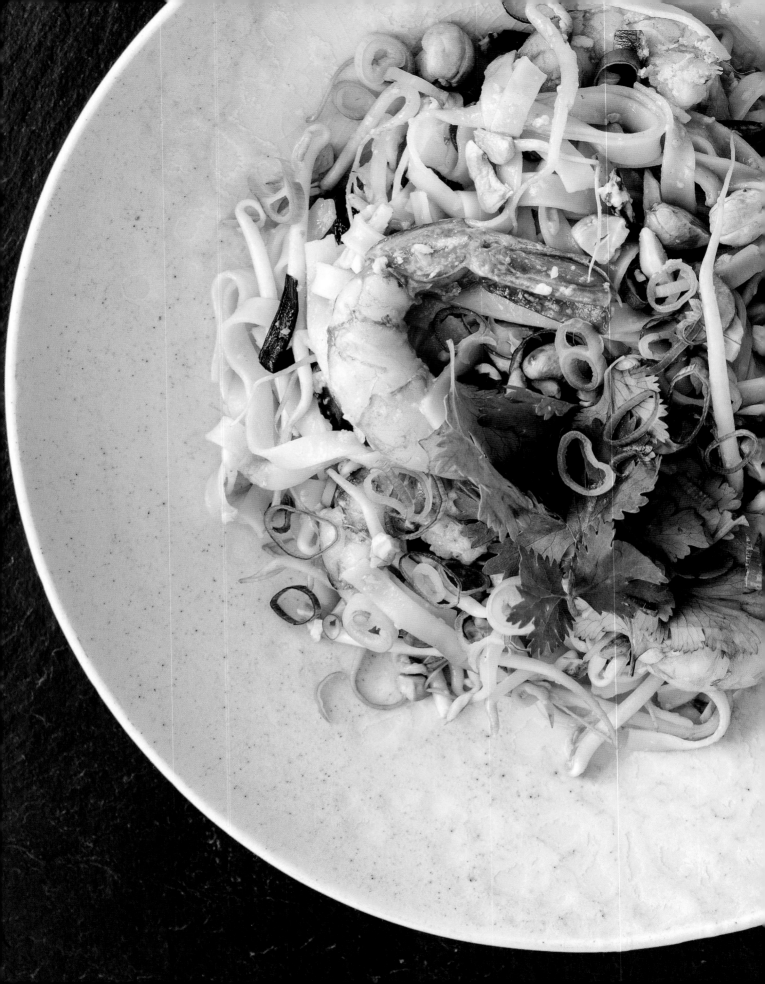

Golden Pad Thai

Place the noodles in a large bowl. Pour boiling water over them, and let them sit to soften up for 1–2 minutes. Stir them occasionally and check them by biting into a strand to ensure that they are tender but not mushy. Peel and slice the garlic thinly. Rinse the spring onions and slice them thinly. Rinse and drain the sprouts. Rinse and pick the coriander. Crack the eggs into a bowl and whisk them together. Season with salt.

In a large wok over medium-high heat, heat up the olive oil. Add the shrimp, garlic and dried chilies, then fry for 1–2 minutes until the shrimp is cooked but not rubbery and dry. Add the eggs and cook for 1 minute. Add the noodles and cook until heated through. Add the spring onions, soy sauce and fish sauce, then stir until just warmed through. Remove the wok from the heat, then season with salt, lime zest and juice to taste. Serve topped with the cashews and coriander.

TIP: This dish can be made with thinly sliced chicken, pork or beef.

400 g pad thai rice noodles

3 cloves garlic

1 bunch fresh spring or green onions

100 g bean sprouts

1 bunch fresh coriander or cilantro

400 g peeled large shrimp

1 pinch crushed dried chilies (optional)

2 whole large eggs

50 mL soy sauce

25 mL fish sauce

Zest and juice of 2 limes

50 g toasted cashews

2 tbsp. olive oil

Salt, to taste

Chicken-quinoa Cobb Salad

Bring the quinoa to a boil in lightly salted water. Reduce the heat to medium-low and cook for 10 minutes. Remove the pot from the heat and let it rest for 5 minutes. Strain the quinoa really well and let it sit in the pot covered until serving. Bring a casserole of salted water to a boil, submerge the eggs, and boil for 6.5 minutes. Cool the eggs down in running cold water, then peel and halve them lengthwise.

Heat up a frying pan with 1 tbsp. of olive oil and fry the sliced ham until crisp. Place the fried pieces on a piece of paper towel. Pick or dice the chicken, then season with salt and pepper. Halve and pit the avocados, scoop the flesh out, and slice it thinly. Rinse and dice the tomatoes, then season with salt and pepper. Cut the romaine lettuce into 3 cm-wide pieces, then rinse and dry them well.

Combine the apple cider vinegar, mustard, honey, salt and pepper, then whisk in the remaining olive oil. Season with salt, pepper and vinegar to taste. Plate all the ingredients side-by-side on top of the quinoa and serve the dressing on the side.

200 g quinoa

4 eggs

4 slices dried ham

400 g leftover chicken or cooked chicken breast

2 avocados

4 large ripe tomatoes

1 head romaine lettuce

2 tbsp. apple cider vinegar

2 tbsp. Dijon mustard

1 tbsp. honey

100 mL olive oil

Salt and pepper, to taste

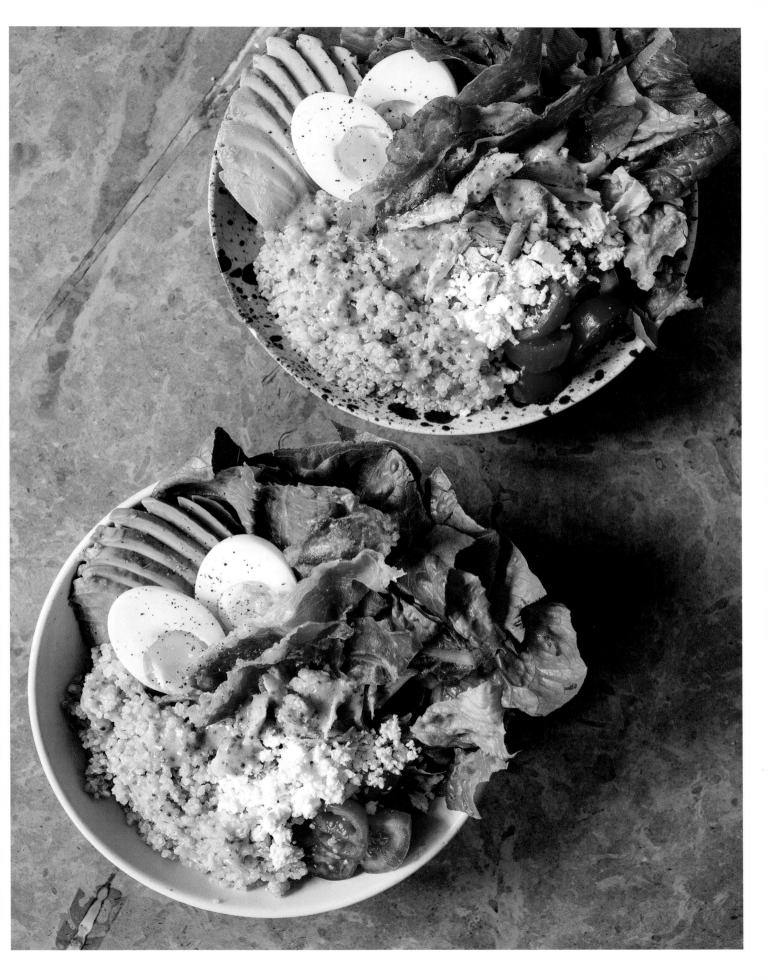

AUTUMN
ERW

Autumn Breakfasts

Autumn Lunches, Dinners and Sides

AUTUMN: OFF-SEASON

As the racing season wraps up, you will need to consider how well your body has coped with a high exercise load all summer long. Your immune system has likely taken a hit as the days get shorter, and you are likely to be more vulnerable to the cold and flu viruses.

The recipes in this section were created to work with your body for total recovery. Many are rich in quercetin: an antioxidant found in onions, grapes, and apples that is particularly good at resisting the flu virus. There are also many dishes that contain allicin: an antioxidant found in garlic, onions, and chives that is also packed with anti-viral properties.

Eat Race Win! Keywords for Autumn

- Breads

- Items that will satisfy your cravings for salty, sweet, fatty, and indulgent foods

- Breakfasts with carbs, proteins, and fats; egg whites, whey, and quinoa are particularly good choices

- Lunches with a nice blend of fats and vegetables

- Dinners with fatty animal proteins - often oven-roasted or braised, legumes, root vegetables, warm spices and herbs

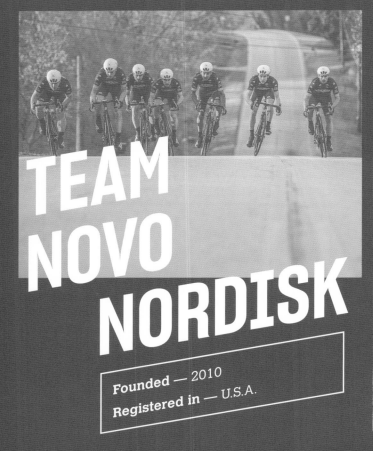

TEAM NOVO NORDISK

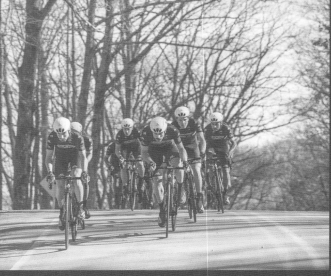

Founded — 2010
Registered in — U.S.A.

Team Novo Nordisk are on a mission to change the way we think about diabetes. Every rider on the squad has Type 1 diabetes and by riding at an elite level, they hope to inspire, empower and educate. I spoke with riders Romain Gioux and Chris Williams, as well as team nutritionist Charlotte Hayes about the role diet and nutrition play in preparing the team to meet the challenges of elite competition.

"With diabetes, nutrition is the cornerstone to management whether you're an athlete or not," Charlotte tells me. "Physical activity, medication, sleeping well, psycho-social support, overall well-being and stress management are all important; but for the team, it's kind of unique because most of them have some sort of foundation in understanding nutrition. We then add an overlay of performance nutrition as well."

She says that Novo Nordisk apply sports nutrition just like any other team, with added adaptations for glucose management and a focus on health and the quality of nutrition. She works with riders on the development squad, reinforcing the right nutritional messages by using visual aids like the US athlete's plate to convey sophisticated concepts like nutrition periodisation in a straightforward way. "It also helps them to understand that foods are your fuel: they help you to recover, feel good, and be healthier."

It's something that Chris Williams understands well. One of the senior riders in the elite squad, the Australian was diagnosed with the disease at 26 after becoming a triathlete when his college girlfriend made an approving comment about the triathlete physique. "I was an overweight smoker, and I told her I could look like that if I wanted to. 3 weeks later, I had quit smoking, sold my car and bought a bike." Eventually focusing on cycling - "I hated swimming and running!"- Chris is one of the squad's super domestiques who believes that a stable routine is important for Type 1 athletes. "I find it a lot easier to control my blood sugar when I ride my bike and eat the same diet every day," he shares, "but you can't have a cheat day because you're really going to feel it trying to control your blood sugar!"

For Romain Gioux, who started on the bike at 8 yet didn't turn professional until he turned 30, good diabetes management has allowed him to change his life and career at a relatively old age for a cyclist. "With maturity, I've been able to make the right nutritional choices," he tells me. "However, the choice is pretty simple - the more I train, the more carbs I eat." It's an approach that Chris echoes. When in training, he eats very low-carb meals, which means that he needs less insulin and has a reduced chance of becoming hypoglycemic or putting on weight. "My carb intake increases when I race, with pasta and rice for fueling." Romain says that on a race day, he eats around 200 grams of carbohydrates to suit his light 50 kg frame, and adds lean chicken for protein.

Charlotte mentions that one of the biggest mistakes she sees in the development squad is the kind of mistake pro riders learn not to make: "Not hydrating enough, not fueling enough, not making a good plan of how many grams of carbohydrates to eat in an hour and how they'll disperse that across the hour." She steers the younger riders away from what she sees as nutritional fads that are not always science-based, instead preferring to encourage her riders to "use the experts who know the science to understand the way it affects their performance."

Talking to the team, it becomes clear that there really isn't a one-size-fits-all approach to nutrition at Novo Nordisk. Chris laughs: "There's no golden rule. Everyone's looking for the rule and it's very different for everyone. I eat virtually no carbs but I have a teammate who practically lives on them! You need to find out what works for you." Romain agrees: "My diabetes has always been pretty well-regulated so I haven't had to change my nutrition in a long time." Both Chris and Romain point out that their diet is no different to any other rider without diabetes. "In my musette, I have paninis with jam or ham and cream cheese, as well as protein bars and sugar-free electrolyte drinks," Chris says, to which Romain agrees, adding: "it is essential to eat healthily to be able to perform at 100% on the bike. The only difference with other athletes is that depending on what I eat, I'll be very vigilant about my sugar levels."

Charlotte pipes in: "The combo of foods is pretty much the same as that of the other teams because our Type 1 athletes are working at the same level of intensity. They're able to use the food as fuel far more effectively than someone who has diabetes and isn't exercising." Refuelling gels and electrolyte drinks are all used by the team, along with energy bars that the team make themselves. Chris points out that he has to be careful about using some engineered solutions like energy gels, as they can cause sugar spikes because they're absorbed so quickly. However, every rider undergoes continuous glucose monitoring using sensors throughout a race, so that their interstitial glucose can be closely observed. "We take a reading every 3-5 minutes," Charlotte says, "and we can see if the glucose is rising or falling so riders can fuel appropriately to sustain their energy output."

Off-season, the team emphasise the need for recovery and preparation for the upcoming season. "We ask our riders to focus on maintaining a healthy weight to stay lean and be able to come into the season where they want to be," Charlotte notes. She helps the development squad riders to understand that no two days are the same, and that they need to adapt their nutrition depending on their circumstances. She also gives them a solid nutritional foundation that is designed to take them from the development squad at 18 to the elite squad by encouraging them to make their own food choices by shopping for and preparing their own food.

What about for the older riders in the squad like Romain and Chris? "At any age, we have to get smarter about nutrition," she replies. "Whether you're fit or not, each decade has different requirements, and health indicators become more challenging to manage. Plus, the effects of a chronic disease can start to add up as we age, so it's really important to be wiser because it can be really challenging to lose that extra kilo or two." Chris agrees, adding, "I can't eat like I used to do at university where I lived on bread, noodles and pasta. If I did that now, I'd put on 10 kg!" He's aware that his metabolism has changed over time, and like Romain, he knows he needs far less fuel in the off-season than he once did. Sidelined with a broken leg for several months, he has tried to keep on top of his calorie intake but admits: "I need to eat healthily but also maintain my sanity!"

"Basically, at any age, diabetic or not, we need to develop great nutritional strategies," Charlotte concludes. "We focus on fruit and vegetables, whole grains and lean proteins; and that's true for all athletes." When it comes to performance nutrition, Charlotte wants her riders to understand nutrition periodization, despite the complications that can arise from insulin matching. "We want our riders to understand when it's time to have more carbs and more carb availability to boost glycogen stores, and when it's a matter of training well to potentially enhance the regulation of enzymes."

By using a combination of technology, diet and continuous glucose monitoring, team Novo Nordisk are using high-performance nutrition to fuel their riders, maintain glucose levels, deliver high-intensity performance, and recover using the same smart sports nutrition strategies that any rider would use. In the process, they're setting the record straight on this often misunderstood condition and changing diabetes with every stroke of the pedal.

"There is no golden rule. Everyone's looking for the rule and it's very different for everyone."

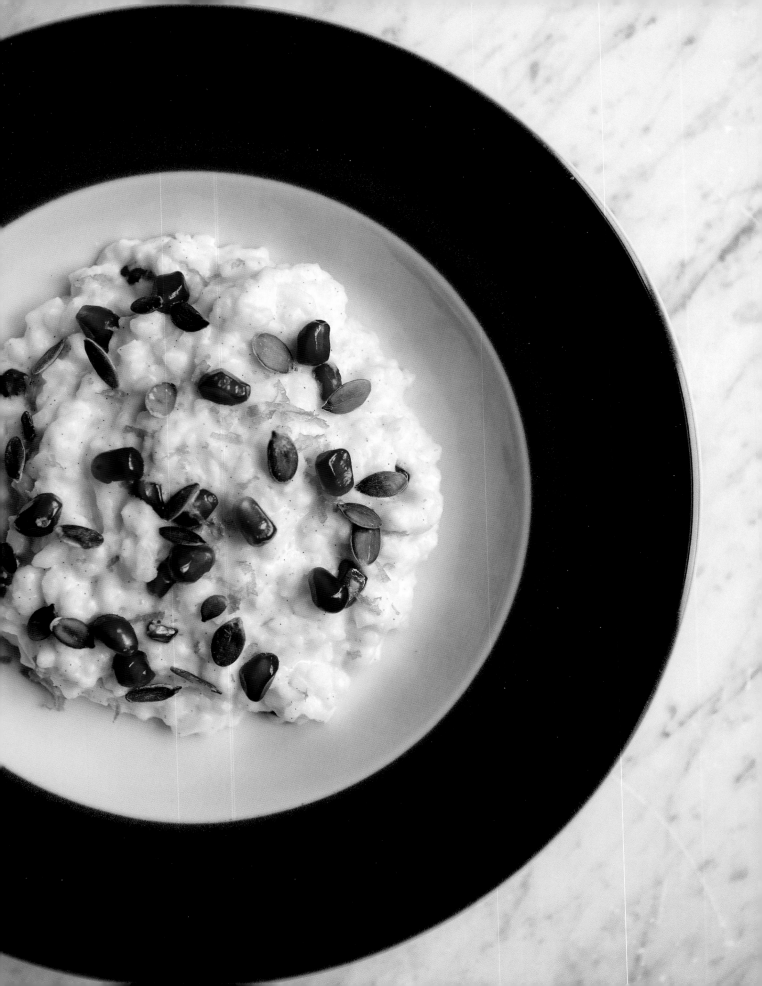

Warm Rice Pudding
with Vanilla, Orange, and Pomegranate

In a pot over medium heat, split the vanilla bean lengthwise and scrape out the seeds. Add the rice and milk, then stirring constantly, slowly bring it to a boil. Reduce the heat to medium-low and let it simmer under a lid for 30–35 minutes, stirring occasionally until the rice grains' cores are soft. Add a splash of water if it gets too dry. Season with orange zest, juice, honey and salt to taste.

⸻

Hold the pomegranate half face down in the palm of your hand over a bowl of water. Hit the top of the pomegranate with the back of a wooden spoon and let the arils fall out into the water. Remove the white membrane and strain the arils. Serve the pudding in deep plates, after topping with the pomegranate, pumpkin seeds and orange zest.

½ vanilla bean

250 mL round rice

1000 mL milk or non-dairy milk

Zest of 1 orange, to taste and serve

Honey, to taste

1 tsp. salt

1 medium pomegranate

30 g pumpkin seeds

Oatmeal with Pear-quince Compote and Cocoa Nibs

Ⓖ Ⓓ Ⓝ Ⓥ

Peel the pear and quince. Quarter them, then cut out and discard the cores. Dice the pear and quince into bite-sized pieces.
In a saucepan over low heat, combine the pear and quince with 50 mL of water. Cover and cook for 15-20 minutes until the consistency is thick and mushy. Remove the pan from the heat and set it aside to cool.

In a large saucepan over medium-high heat, bring 800 mL water and the salt to a boil. Whisk in the oats and bring it to a boil. Reduce the heat to medium-low and simmer, stirring occasionally for 10 minutes, until the oats are fully cooked. Adjust the thickness of the oatmeal to the desired consistency by adding water if needed. Season with salt and honey. Serve in deep plates, after topping with the pear and quince compote as well as a sprinkle of cocoa nibs.

TIP: To add protein, let the oatmeal cool down for about 2 minutes, then whisk an egg into it. The oatmeal should not be reheated after the egg has been added.

1 medium pear

1 medium quince

850 mL water, divided

½ tsp. salt

200 g rolled oats

Honey, to taste

10 g cocoa nibs

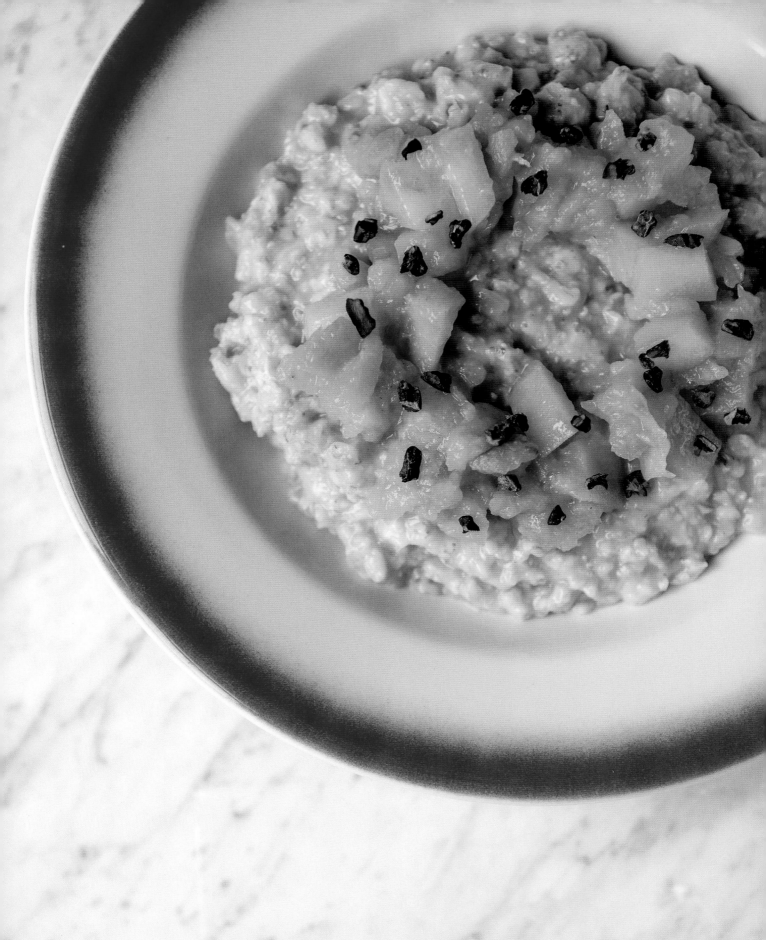

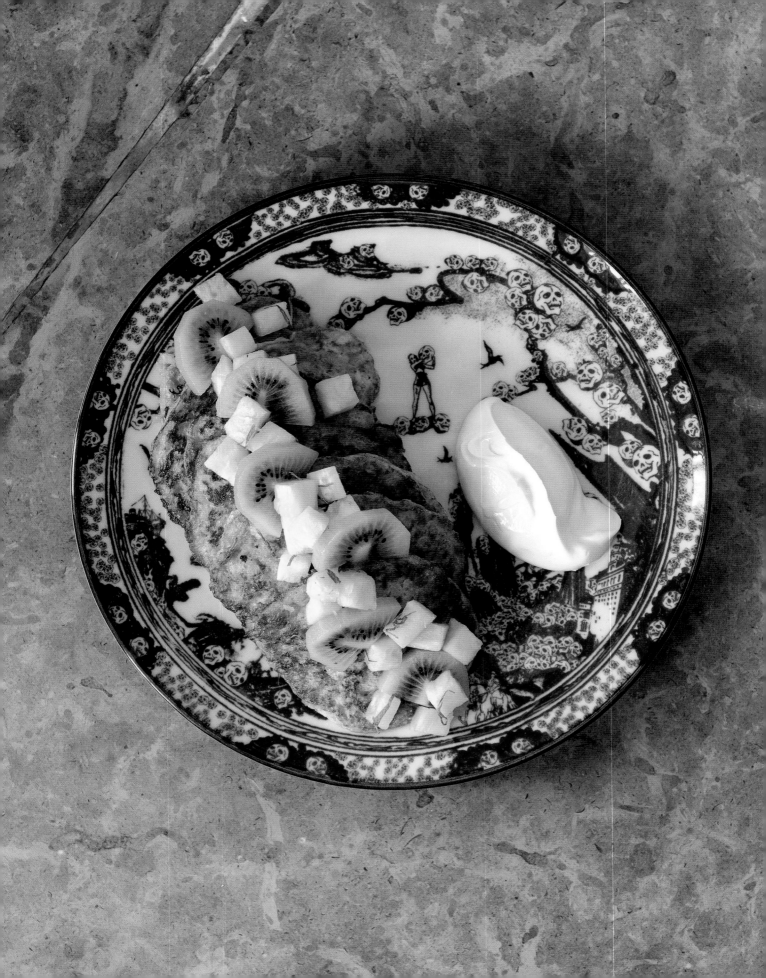

Oatmeal Pancakes with Pineapple and Kiwi Fruit

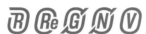

In a large mixing bowl, combine the cooked oatmeal, eggs, sugar, lemon zest, salt and cardamom. Stir until well combined. In a frying pan over medium heat, heat up the olive oil. Add 3 small spoons of the batter and cook for 2 minutes on each side until golden and firm. Transfer the pancakes onto a plate and cover with tin foil to keep warm. Repeat this process until all of the batter has been used, then remove the pan from the heat.

———

Cut off the rind of the pineapple and dice the fruit into cubes. Peel and slice the kiwi fruit. Serve the pancakes topped with fruit and yogurt on the side.

500 g cooked oatmeal

2 whole large eggs

15 g sugar

Zest of 1 lemon

1 pinch salt

1 pinch cardamom

3 tbsp. olive oil

¼ pineapple

2 kiwis

250 mL plain Greek yogurt

Soft Polenta with Oranges, Cinnamon, Cranberries, and Almonds

In a saucepan over medium-high heat, bring the water and salt to a boil. Whisk in the polenta. Reduce the heat to low and cook, stirring constantly for 5 minutes until the polenta is smooth. Cover the pan, remove it from the heat, and set it aside.

—

Rinse and dry the oranges, then finely grate them for their zest. Using a sharp knife, cut off the oranges' tops and bottoms. Carefully cut off the rinds from the top towards the bottom; removing the white membrane and as little orange flesh as possible. Slice the flesh into wedges by sliding the knife down next to the membrane on each side and letting the pulp fall into a bowl. Remove all the seeds.

—

Heat up the polenta and adjust the texture to your liking with a splash of water. Add the almonds, then season with the orange zest and maple or date syrup to taste. Add more salt if needed. Remove the pan from the heat. Serve the polenta in bowls topped with the cranberries and orange salad on the side.

—

TIP: If you are training, mix the cranberries into the polenta and pour it into a container lined with parchment paper. Let it cool down completely in the refrigerator, then slice into squares to wrap and bring along for a training pass or lunch.

1000 mL water
1 tsp. salt
150 g polenta
1 orange
1 blood orange
100 g finely chopped almonds
Maple/date syrup, to taste
Fresh mint leaves
50 g dried cranberries

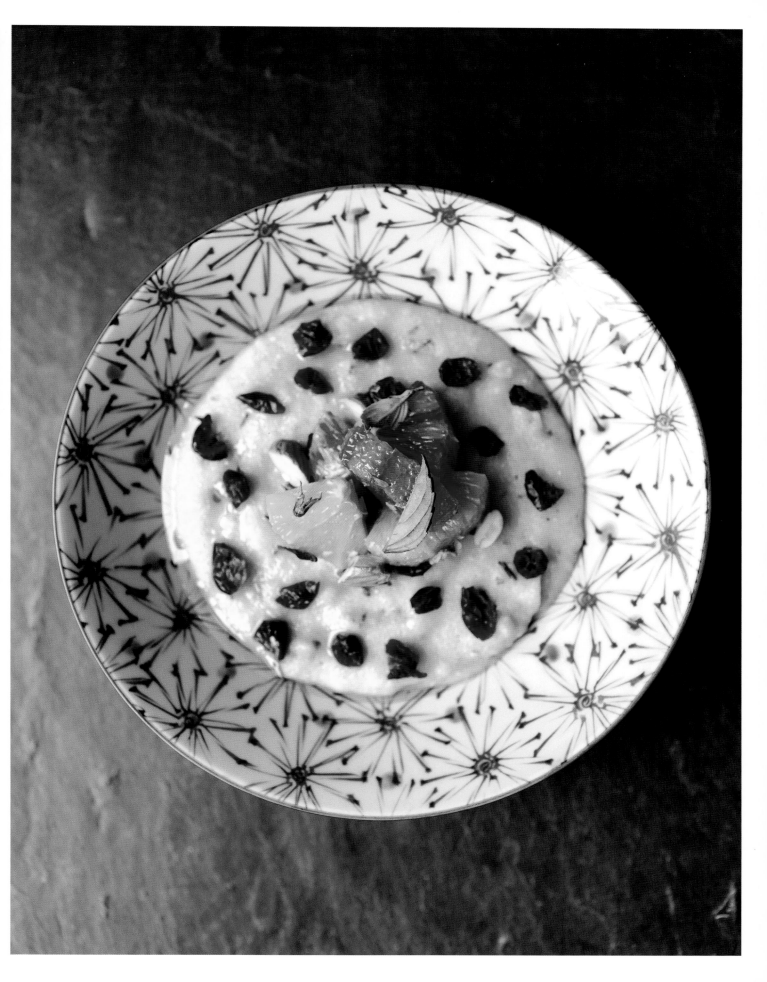

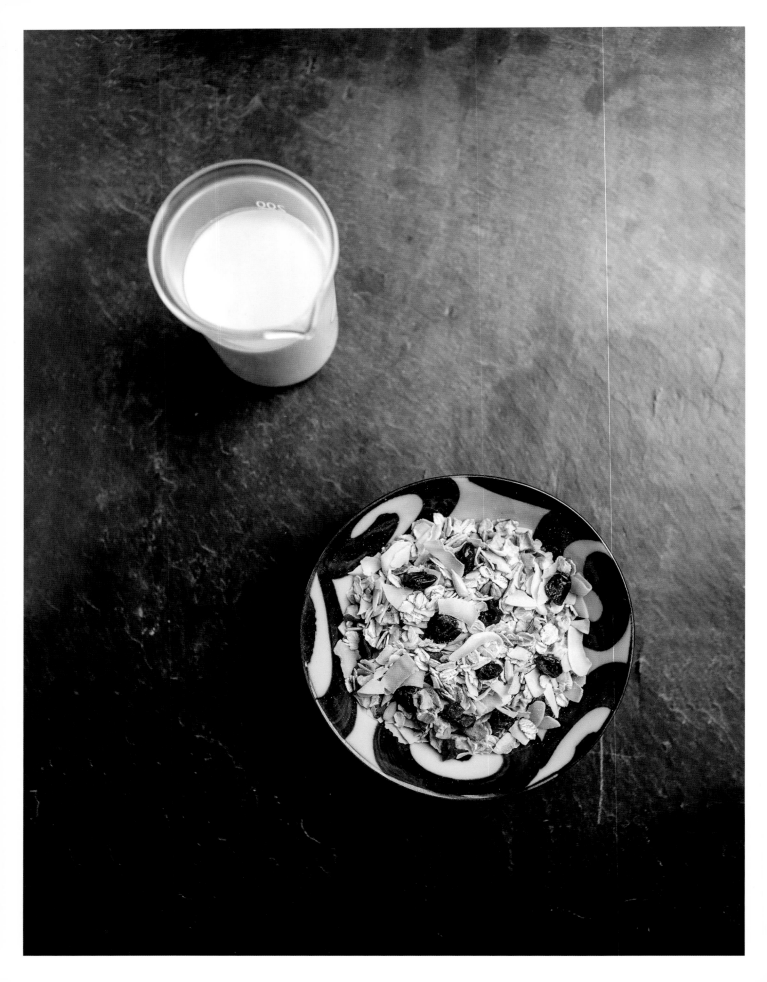

Toasted Coconut Müesli

Preheat the oven to 175°C/350°F. Line a baking sheet with parchment paper. Place the coconut on the prepared sheet and toast for about 10–12 minutes until golden. For an extra-toasty flavor, toast the oats as well. Remove the sheet from the oven and set it aside to cool. In an airtight container, combine the cooled coconut, oats, dried apples, cherries or cranberries, and all the seeds. Shake to ensure that the mixture is well combined, then serve.

100 g shredded or shaved coconut

500 g rolled oats

100 g diced dried apples

50 g dried cherries or cranberries

50 g pumpkin seeds

50 g sunflower seeds

Seasonal sliced fruit, to serve

Overnight Müesli

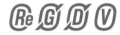

Combine all the ingredients and refrigerate the mixture overnight. Serve for breakfast or as part of a recovery meal.

200 g toasted coconut müesli

400 mL non-dairy milk

100 g diced fresh fruit or shredded carrot

Non-dairy / Plant-based Milk

Soak the almonds in cold water with 1 pinch of salt for 8–12 hours or overnight. Strain the almonds, then blend them with fresh water, your desired spices, and 1 pinch of salt until smooth. Strain and squeeze the liquid through a piece of cheesecloth. Refrigerate it in a clean bottle or container for up to 4 days.

SOAKING TIME FOR OTHER NUTS

Hazelnuts: 8 hours

Macadamias: 8 hours

Peanuts: 8 hours

Pecans: 4-6 hours

Walnuts: 4 hours

Cashews: 2 hours

Brazil Nuts: No soaking needed

TIP: You can dry the nut pulp in a dehydrator or the oven at 150°C/300°F, then pulse it in a food processor to make nut flour.

10 ▌ — 12 ▌

For almond milk:

250 g finely chopped almonds

1000 mL water

Salt, to taste

Vanilla bean, ground cinnamon and honey, to taste (optional)

Oat Milk

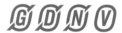

Soak the oats in water with salt for 15 minutes. Blend the mixture until smooth. Strain and squeeze the liquid through a piece of cheesecloth. Refrigerate in a clean bottle or container for up to 5 days.

If using a high speed blender, make sure the oats don't cook as you blend.

100 g rolled oats

1000 mL water

1 pinch of salt

Vanilla bean, ground cinnamon, and honey, to taste (optional)

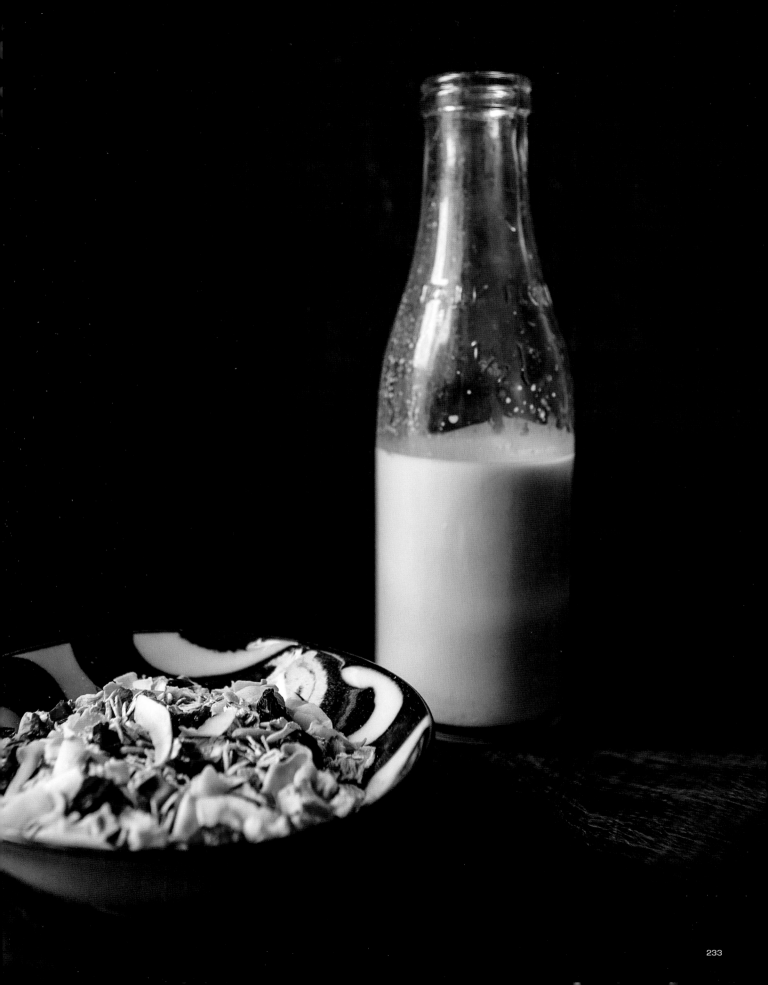

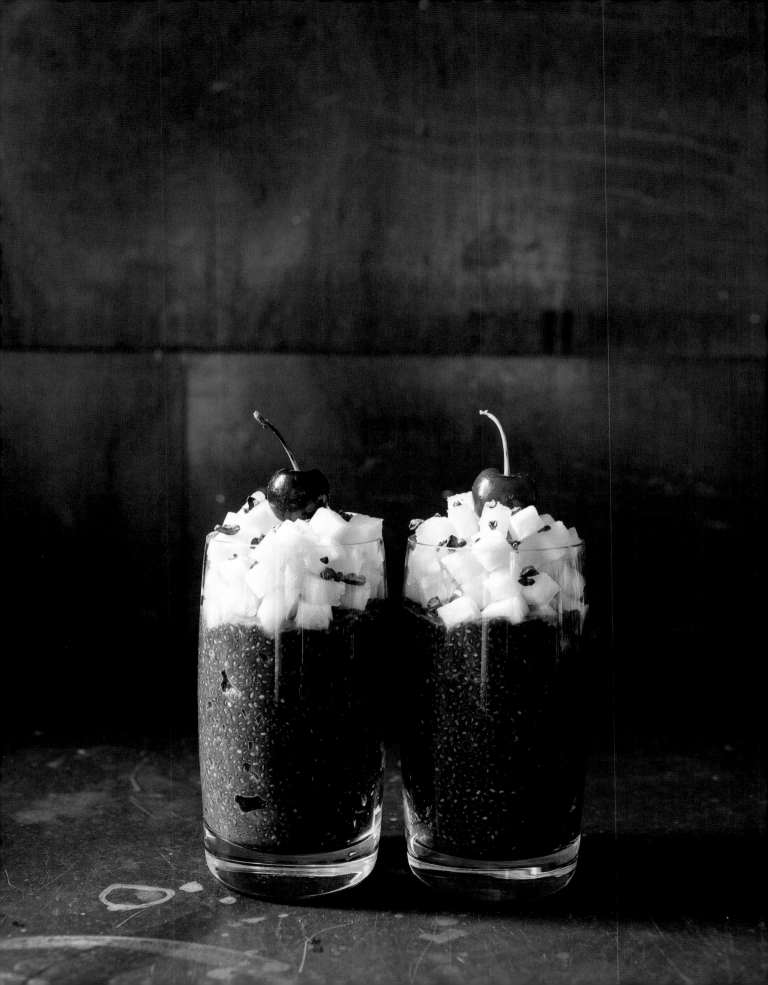

Cocoa Chia Pudding with Pineapple

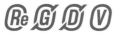

Combine the chia seeds, cocoa powder and non–dairy milk. Season with salt and maple or date syrup, then refrigerate for at least 4 hours or overnight in your desired serving bowls. Dice the pineapple. Serve the chia pudding topped with the pineapple and cocoa nibs for breakfast, as a recovery meal, or for dessert.

50 g chia seeds

3 tbsp. unsweetened cocoa powder

300 mL non-dairy milk (see recipe on p.232)

1 pinch of salt

Maple/date syrup, to taste

¼ pineapple

1 tsp. cocoa nibs

Oatmeal Bannocks
with Blackberries and Greek Yogurt

Preheat the oven to 205°C/400°F. Line a baking sheet with parchment paper. In a large mixing bowl, combine the dry ingredients. Crumble the butter into the mixture by hand. Add the water and gather the rough dough together to knead briefly. Carefully roll out the dough into a 5 mm–thick sheet, then punch or cut out circles. Place them on the prepared sheet and mark a cross on the top of each circle with a knife. Bake for about 20 minutes until golden. Remove them from the oven and serve them warm, topped with yogurt, blackberries and honey to taste.

250 g rolled oats

250 g oat flour

¼ tsp. salt

55 g butter, diced

120 mL water

100 mL plain Greek yogurt, to serve

100 g fresh blackberries, to serve

Honey, to taste

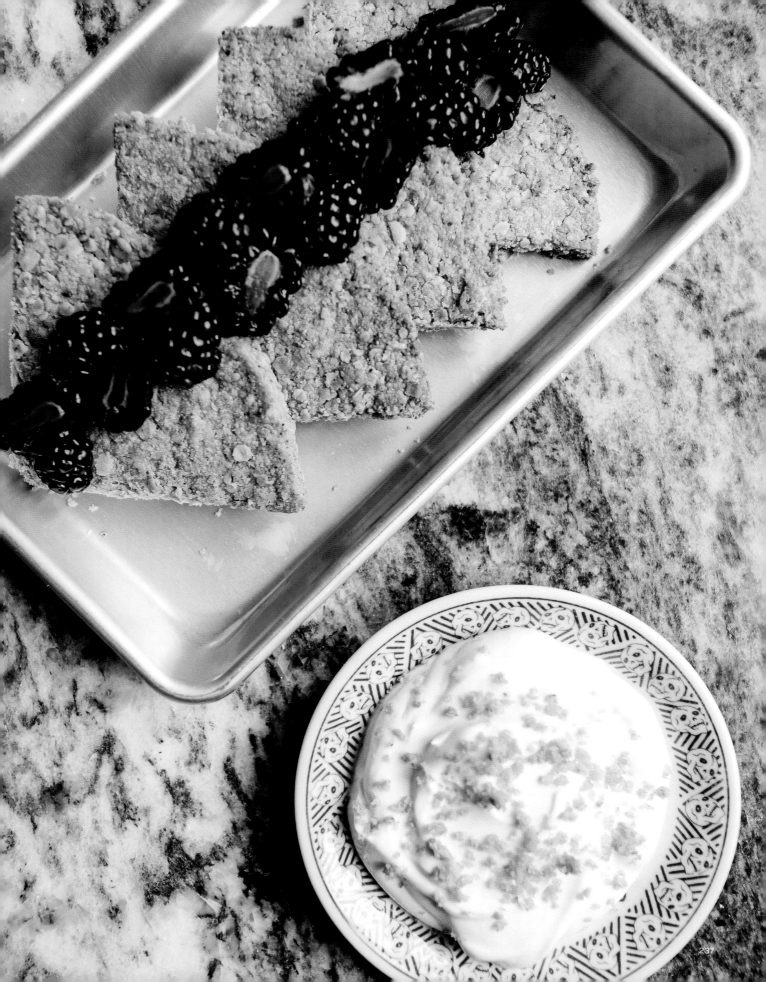

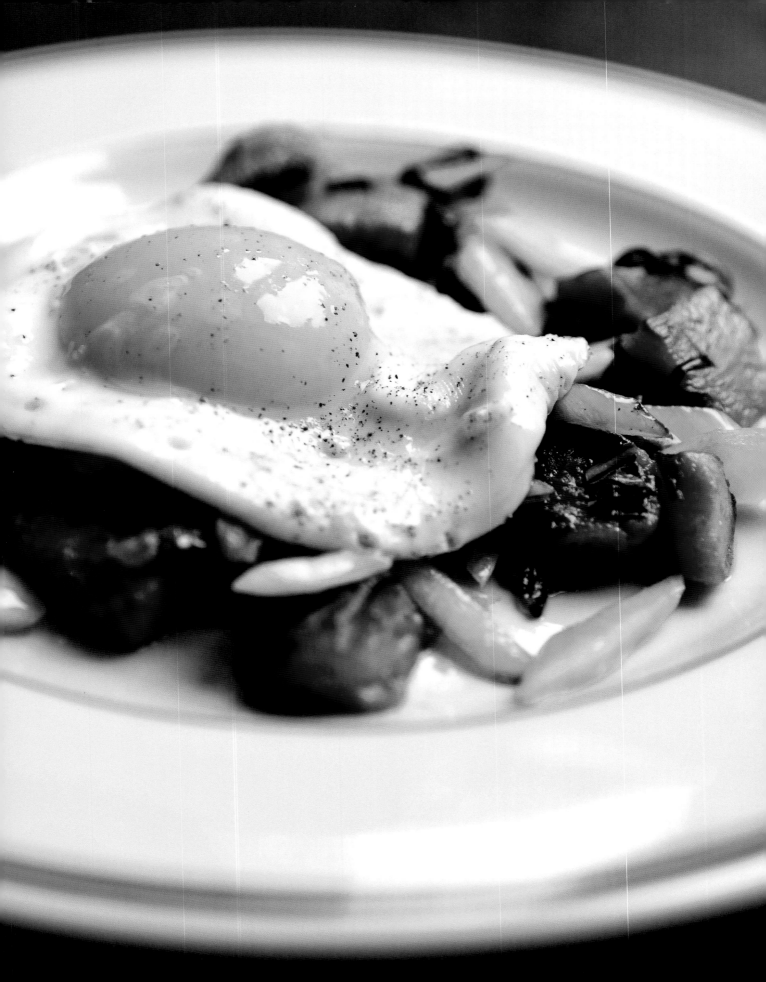

Sweet Potato Hash
with Bok Choy and Fried Eggs

Re G D V

Preheat the oven to 185°C/365°F. Line a baking sheet with parchment paper. Scrub or peel the sweet potatoes and dice them into bite-sized pieces. Place them onto the prepared sheet and bake for about 25-30 minutes until they are soft in the center. Remove them from the oven.

Rinse and cut the bok choy into bite-sized diagonal pieces. Peel and slice the garlic. Heat up a frying pan with 2 tbsp. of oil and roast the sweet potatoes until golden brown. Add the garlic and bok choy, then sauté for 2 minutes until the bok choy is vivid green and tender. Season with salt and pepper to taste.

Wipe the pan clean with a paper towel and heat it up over medium-high heat with 1 tbsp. of olive oil. Fry the eggs until the egg white has set and the yolk is still runny. Arrange the sweet potatoes and bok choy on a plate in the center, then top with the fried egg. Season with salt and pepper.

TIP: You can easily bake a larger batch of sweet potatoes and refrigerate them for a couple of days to serve as a quick breakfast.

2 medium sweet potatoes, rinsed, scrubbed and dried

1 medium head bok choy

1 clove garlic

3 tbsp. olive oil, divided

Salt and pepper, to taste

2 whole large eggs

Köfte, Baked Pumpkin, and Herb Salad with Yogurt Dressing

Preheat the oven to 175°C/350°F. Line 2 baking sheets with parchment paper. Halve the pumpkin and discard the seeds. Place the pumpkin onto a baking sheet and drizzle with 2 tbsp. of oil, then season with salt and pepper. Bake for about 35–40 minutes until the flesh is tender. Remove it from the oven and turn the heat up to 200°C/395°F.

——

Rinse and pick the parsley. Pat it dry with a paper towel and chop ½ of the bunch finely. Set the rest aside for serving. Peel and mince the garlic. Zest and juice the lemons, then set them aside separately. In a large mixing bowl, combine the ground beef, finely chopped parsley, some lemon zest and crushed cloves. Mix by hand until well combined. Season the mixture with salt and pepper, then shape it into egg-shaped meatballs. Place the meatballs onto the second prepared sheet and bake for 8–10 minutes until they are firm. Remove them from the oven.

——

In a small mixing bowl, season the yogurt with some lemon juice, the garlic, salt, and pepper to taste. Sprinkle with chili powder. Toss the picked parsley with 1 tbsp. of olive oil and the remaining lemon juice, then place it on the meatballs. Serve the pumpkin, meatballs and yogurt in separate bowls at the table.

——

TIP: To add carbs, serve a bowl of freshly cooked quinoa, rice or flatbread on the side.

1 medium Hokkaido pumpkin
3 tbsp. olive oil
1 bunch fresh flat-leaf parsley
2 cloves garlic
2 medium lemons
500 g ground beef
1 pinch crushed cloves
250 g plain Greek yogurt
1 pinch mild chili powder
Salt and pepper, to taste

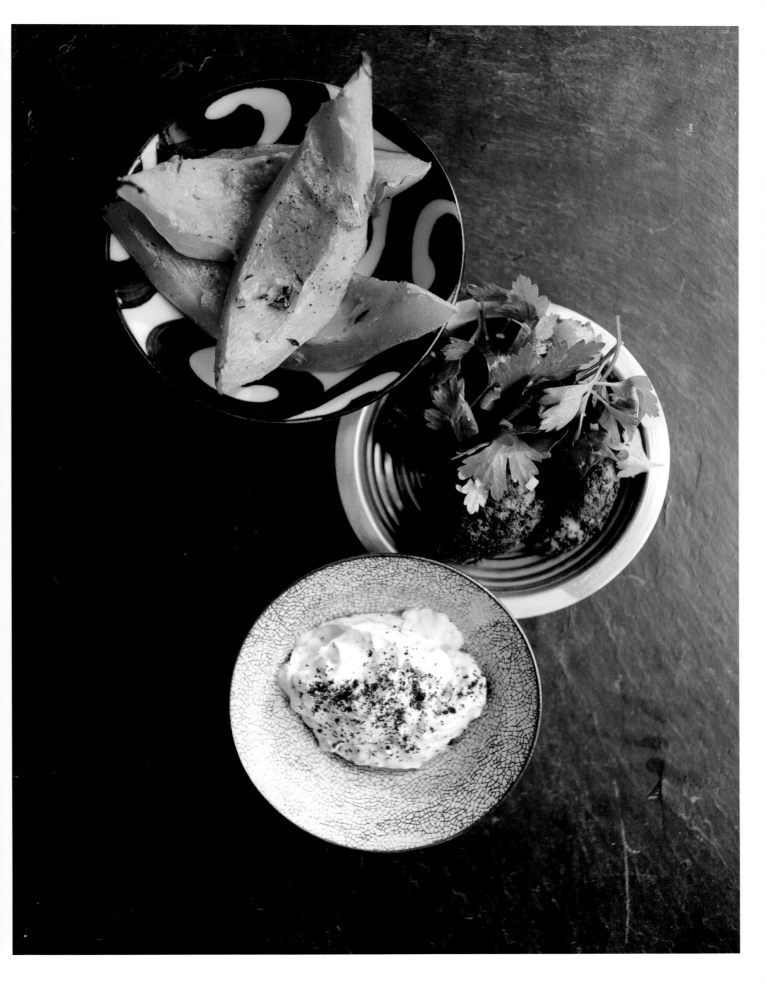

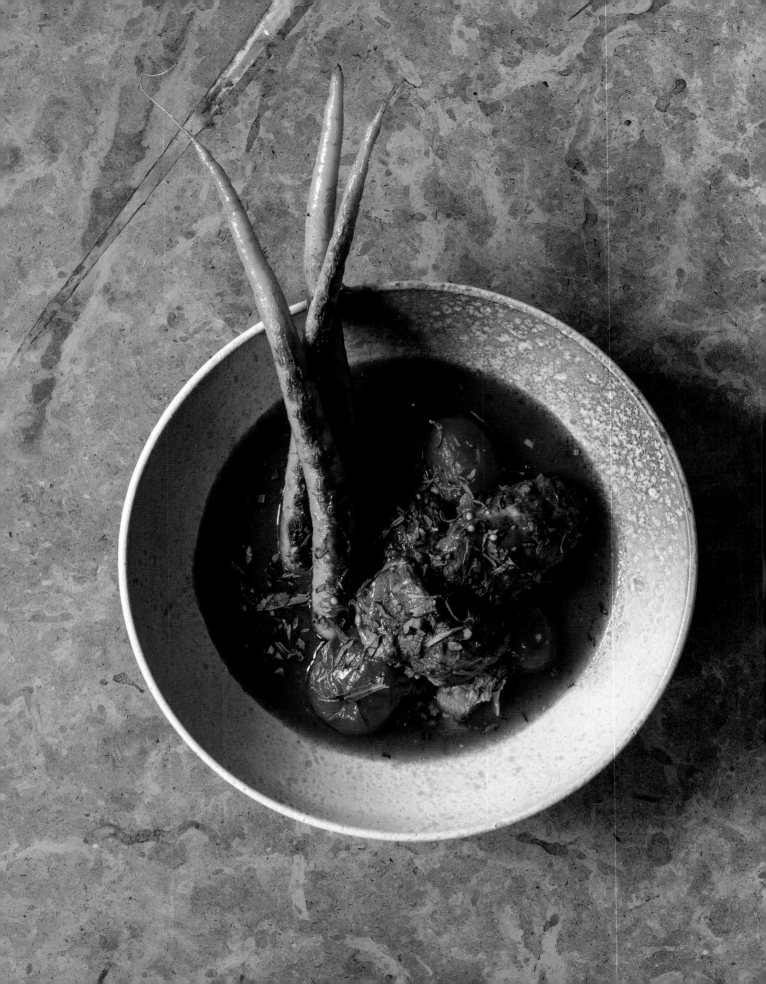

Slow-cooked Pork Cheeks and Tomato in Red Wine

Preheat the oven to 150°C/350°F. Trim the pork cheeks, and remove all bone bits and tendons. Scrub the carrots and split the thickest of them lengthwise. Rinse the tomatoes and halve the head of garlic across the center. Fill a single-use teabag or a piece of cheesecloth with the dried spices and tie it with string.

Transfer the pork cheeks, vegetables and dried spices onto an ovenproof pan. Pour all the liquids into the pan and cover it with tin foil before placing it in the oven to cook for 3 hours.

Remove the tin foil and cook for another 30 minutes to let the sauce reduce down. Remove the teabag and carefully strain the liquid into a saucepan. Set the pork cheeks and vegetables aside, covered with tin foil. Reduce the liquid to about half, then season with salt, pepper and balsamic vinegar. Pour the sauce back over the pork cheeks and vegetables, then garnish them with the fresh tarragon. Serve with the crushed potatoes or polenta.

TIP: To thicken the sauce, whisk 1 tbsp. of cornstarch mixed with 2 tbsp. of cold water into the sauce and bring to a boil for 1-2 minutes until the sauce is thick and smooth.

12 pork cheeks

10-12 whole medium carrots

400 g plum tomatoes

1 head garlic

1 single-use tea bag

5 bay leaves

1 tsp. fennel seeds

1 tsp. coriander seeds

½ tsp. black pepper corns

½ tsp. cloves

1 tsp. salt

400 mL red wine

200 mL water

4 tbsp. balsamic vinegar + more to taste

3 tbsp. honey

1 bunch fresh tarragon

Salt and pepper, to taste

Crushed potatoes or polenta, to serve

The World's Easiest Steamed and Roasted Vegetables

This recipe is possibly the easiest and most delicious way to cook vegetables with very little effort, and you only need 1 pan! Inspired by my daily life, it is also a perfect way to get rid of all the stray and lonely vegetables hanging around in your refrigerator.

ii – iiii

½ celery root

½ cauliflower

4 cloves garlic

Thyme sprigs

2 tbsp. olive oil or butter

Salt, to taste

G N V

Rinse or peel all the vegetables, then cut them into equal-sized chunks. On a cold pan, drizzle the olive oil, sprinkle some salt, and place all the vegetables with the cut side facing down. Cover the pan with a lid and place it over medium heat. Let the vegetables steam/roast in their own released liquids for 10–12 minutes until tender and golden brown. The bigger your pieces are, the longer the cooking time. If so, flip the vegetables over and steam/roast for another 4–5 minutes. Serve as an accompaniment to your desired protein and carb, or use them in frittatas.

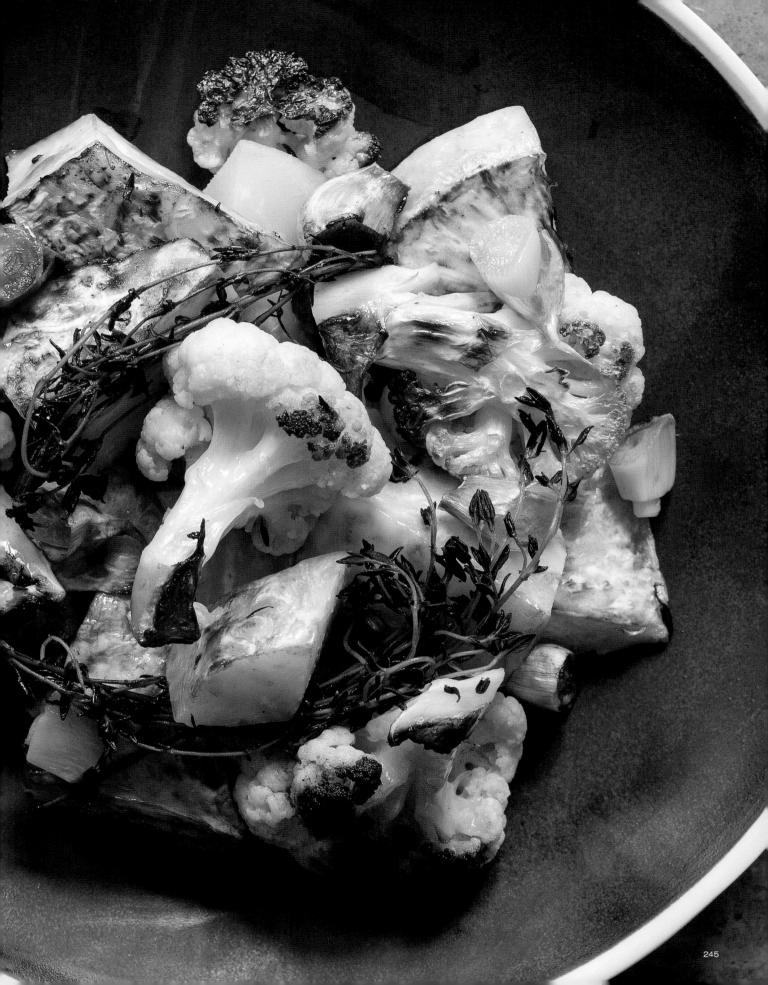

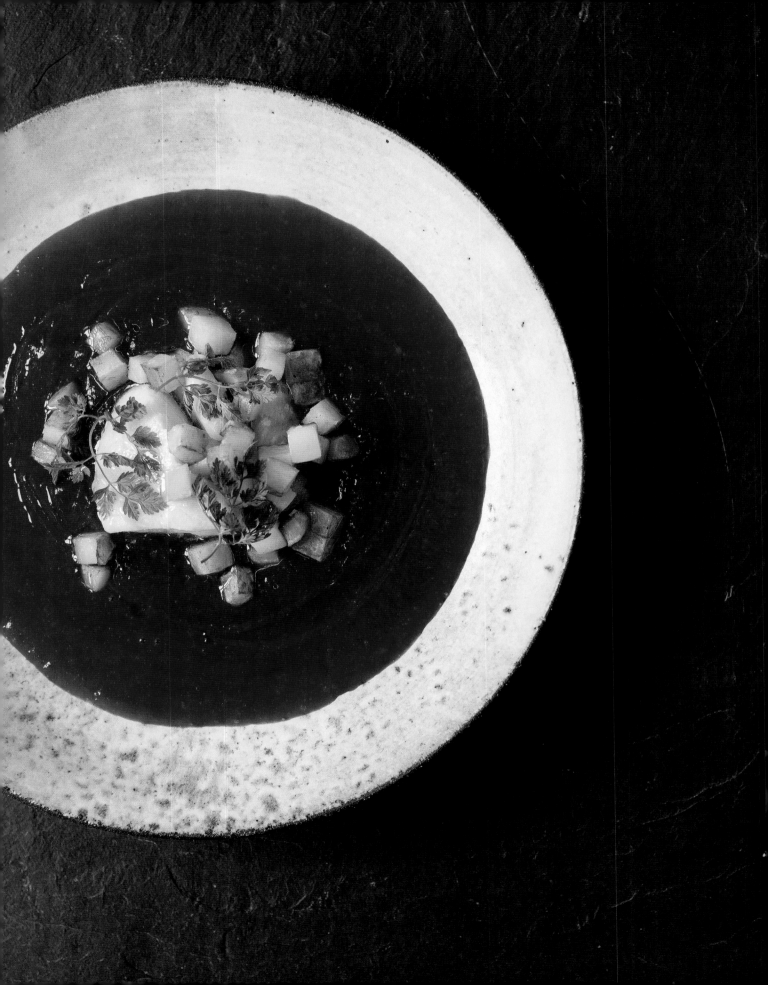

Beet Soup with Baked Cod and Greek Yogurt

Peel the carrots and beets, then cut them into large cubes. Peel the potato and slice half of it into large cubes and the other half into small dices to be used as garnish. Peel and mince the onions, garlic and ginger. In a large pot, sauté the onions, garlic and ginger over medium heat in 1 tbsp. of olive oil until the onions are soft and translucent. Add the beets, carrots, and large potato cubes to the pot. Add the broth and bring it to a boil. Reduce the heat to medium-low and simmer for 30–35 minutes until all the vegetables are tender. Blend all the ingredients until smooth. Pour the soup back into the pot and bring it to a boil again over medium heat, skimming away impurities from the surface. Season with salt, pepper, lime zest and juice to taste.

———

Preheat the oven to 175°C/345°F. Line a baking sheet with parchment paper. Divide the fish into 4 equal-sized pieces and sprinkle them with salt. Place them onto the prepared sheet and bake for about 8–10 minutes until a cake tester slides through the flesh with no resistance. Heat up a small pan with 1 tbsp. of olive oil, sprinkle the pan with salt, then fry the small potato dices until golden brown and tender. Serve the soup in deep plates with a piece of fish at the center. Top with the fried potatos and chervil.

———

TIP: Add cooked lentils, rice or quinoa to the soup to make it a full main course.

300 g carrots

600 g beets

1 large baking potato

2 medium onions

3 cloves garlic

25 g fresh ginger

Olive oil, to cook

1 L chicken or vegetable broth

Zest and juice of 2 limes

400 g fresh skinned cod fillet

4 tbsp. plain Greek yogurt

1 bunch fresh chervil (or other fresh herb)

Salt and pepper, to taste

Chicken Tagine with Sweet Potatoes and Apricots

G D N

Divide the chicken into 8 pieces by separating the upper and lower thighs, and dividing the breast into 4 pieces. Mince the fresh turmeric, ginger, and garlic. In a large mixing bowl, combine them with the cumin, paprika, salt and pepper. Wash, zest and juice the lemons. Add ⅔ of the juice to a large mixing bowl. Place the chicken in it and set it aside to marinate for at least 20 minutes or overnight in the refrigerator. Peel the sweet potatoes and onions. Rinse the peppers. Slice the potatoes into bite-sized pieces. Quarter the onions and halve the dried apricots.

In a tagine or a large Dutch oven over medium-high heat, warm 2 tbsp. of olive oil and brown all the chicken skin without burning it. Add the vegetables, apricots and lemon zest to the tagine. Pour the broth over the mixture and bring it to a boil. Reduce the heat to medium-low, then season with salt and pepper. Simmer it covered for 30-35 minutes until the chicken is fully cooked and tender. Remove the lid and reduce the sauce for another 5-7 minutes. Season with salt, pepper and lemon juice to taste. Serve the chicken in bowls topped with fresh coriander and mint.

TIP: To add more carbs, serve the chicken with steamed rice, couscous or chickpeas.

1 whole chicken

15 g fresh or 3 tbsp. dried turmeric

25 g fresh ginger

4 cloves garlic

½ tbsp. ground cumin

½ tbsp. ground paprika

3 lemons

500 g sweet potatoes

2 red onions

2 red peppers

50 g dried apricots

Olive oil, to cook

500 mL water or broth

½ bunch fresh coriander or cilantro

15 fresh mint leaves

Salt and pepper, to taste

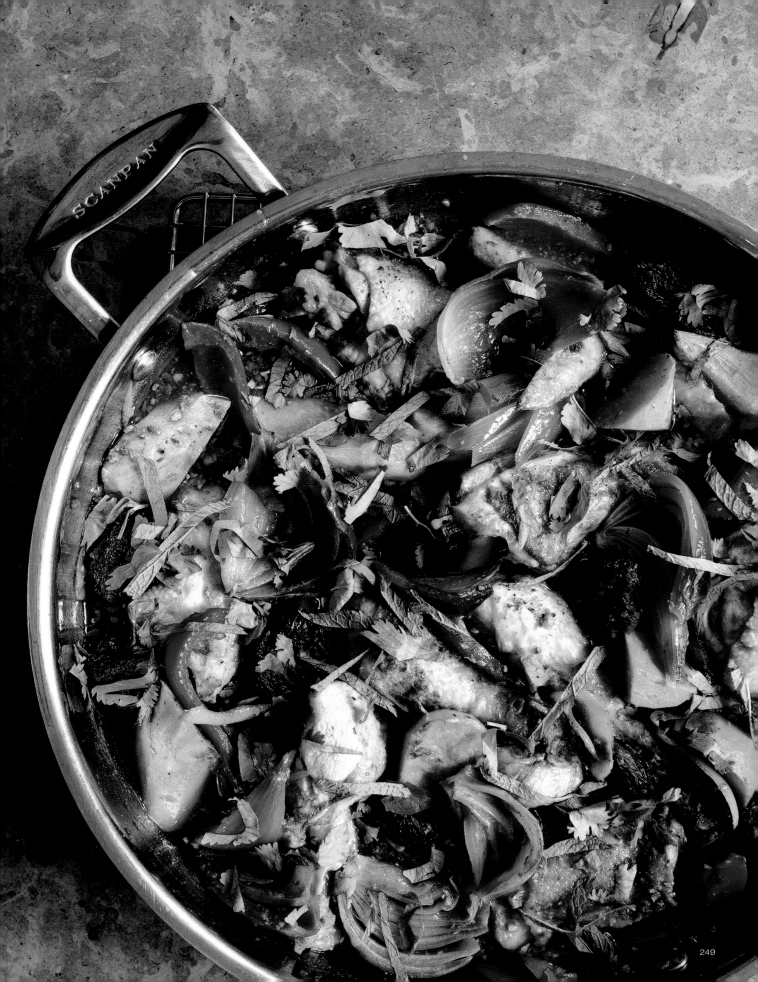

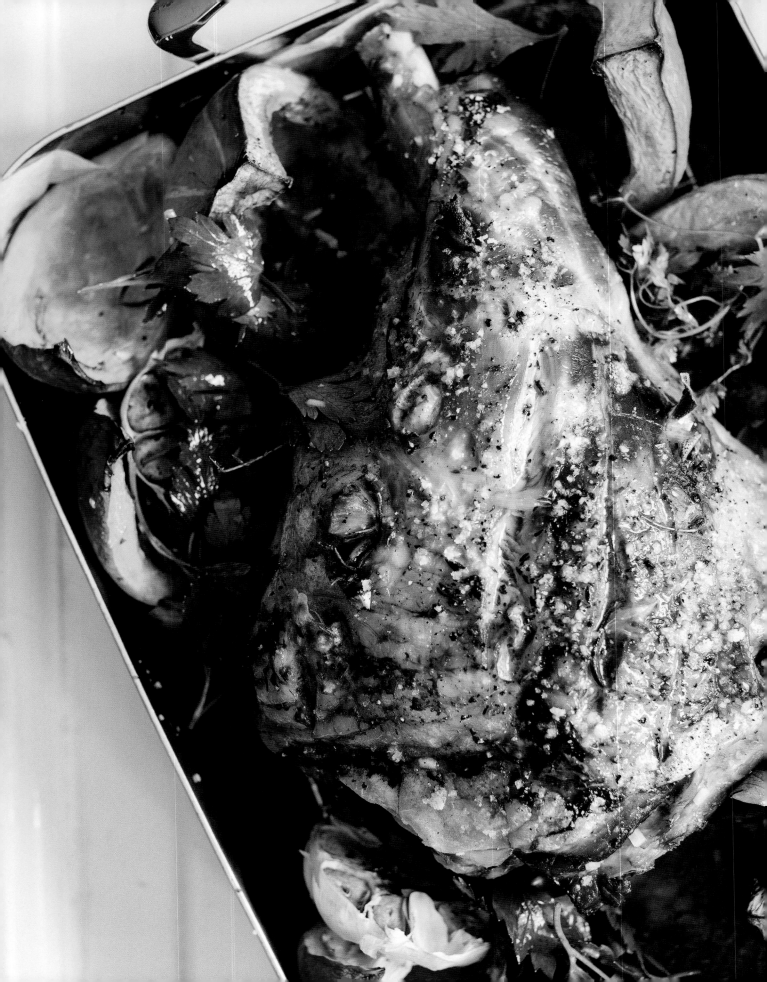

Lamb with Pumpkin, Garlic, and Rosemary

Preheat the oven to 150°C/300°F. Peel 5 cloves of garlic and slice them thinly. Zest the lemons and separate the rosemary leaves from the stems, then discard the stems. In a small mixing bowl, combine the sliced garlic, lemon zest and rosemary leaves. Halve the remaining garlic heads and the zested lemons. Halve the pumpkins and discard the seeds. Brush each pumpkin half with olive oil, then season with salt and pepper.

———

Trim all the thick excess fat from the lamb. Using a paring knife, pierce holes in the lamb and stuff them with the garlic, lemon zest and rosemary mixture. Rub the surface of the lamb with salt and pepper, then drizzle it with olive oil. Place the lamb on top of the pumpkin in a roasting pan. Pierce it with a heatproof meat thermometer in the thickest part, making sure that the tip slides down next to the bone. Arrange the halved garlic heads and halved lemons around the lamb. Roast until the lamb has reached a core temperature of 54°C/130°F or higher, if desired. Remove it from the oven and set it aside to rest for at least 15 minutes before slicing. To serve, scatter the picked parsley around the sliced lamb with crushed potatoes or polenta on the side.

3 heads garlic

2 medium lemons

3 sprigs fresh rosemary

2 small Hokkaido pumpkins

Olive oil, to cook

1 (3.5 kg) leg of lamb

1 bunch fresh flat-leaf parsley

Salt and pepper, to taste

Crushed potatoes or polenta, to serve

Chicken Soup with Brown Rice and Lemon Thyme

Preheat the oven to 225°C/440°F. Salt the chicken and place it in a roasting pan, breast-side down. Roast for 30 minutes, flip it over, and roast for another 7 minutes. Remove it from the oven and set it aside to rest for at least 15 minutes, breast-side down.

———

Rinse and tie ½ the thyme and rosemary twigs together with twine. Add it to the broth in a large stockpot and bring it to a boil slowly. Peel the carrots, rinse the zucchini, and cut them both into small dices. Slice the leeks thinly and rinse them well in cold water, ensuring that all the sand has been washed out. Rinse, pick and chop the parsley finely. Pick the remaining ½ of the thyme and set it aside for serving.

———

When the chicken has cooled down, pick the meat off it and set it aside. Reserve the carcass for future broth. Remove the thyme and rosemary from the broth, then add the leeks, carrots and zucchini. Let it simmer for 1 minute, then add the rice and chicken.
Slowly heat it through, then season with salt, pepper, lemon zest and juice. Serve the chicken in soup bowls topped with the fresh parsley, thyme and Parmesan.

1 (1.4 kg) whole fresh chicken or picked chicken

½ bunch thyme

3 twigs rosemary

1000 mL chicken broth

2 carrots

2 zucchini squash

3 leeks

½ bunch fresh flat-leaf parsley

400 g leftover rice or quinoa

2 lemons

Salt and pepper, to taste

Freshly grated Parmesan cheese, to serve

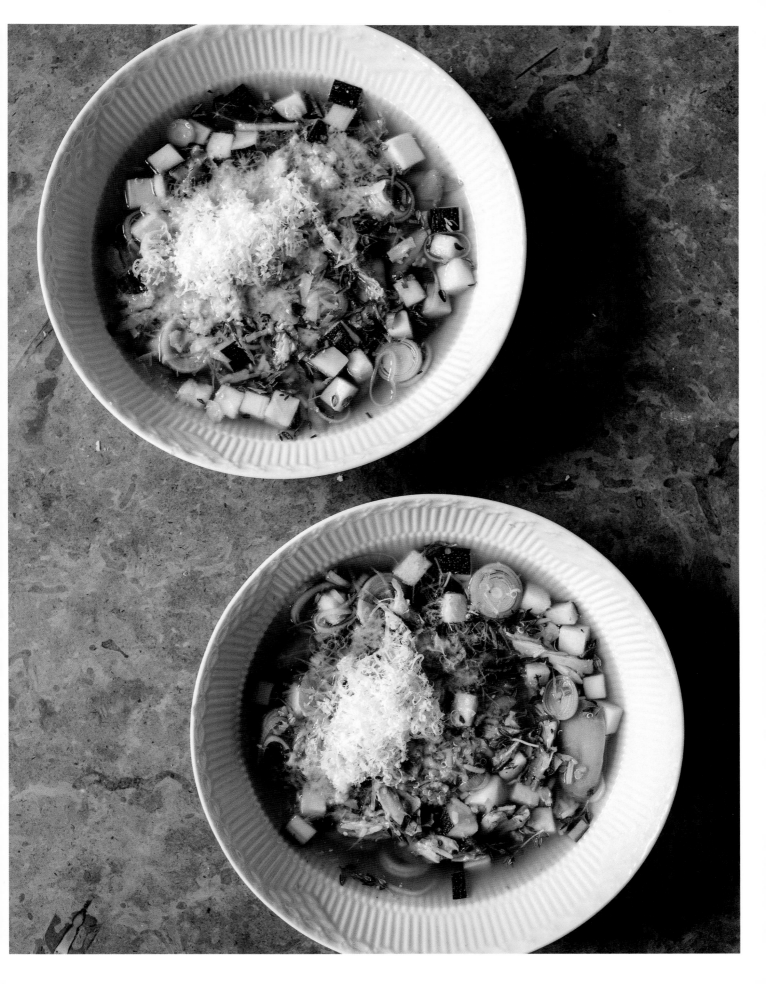

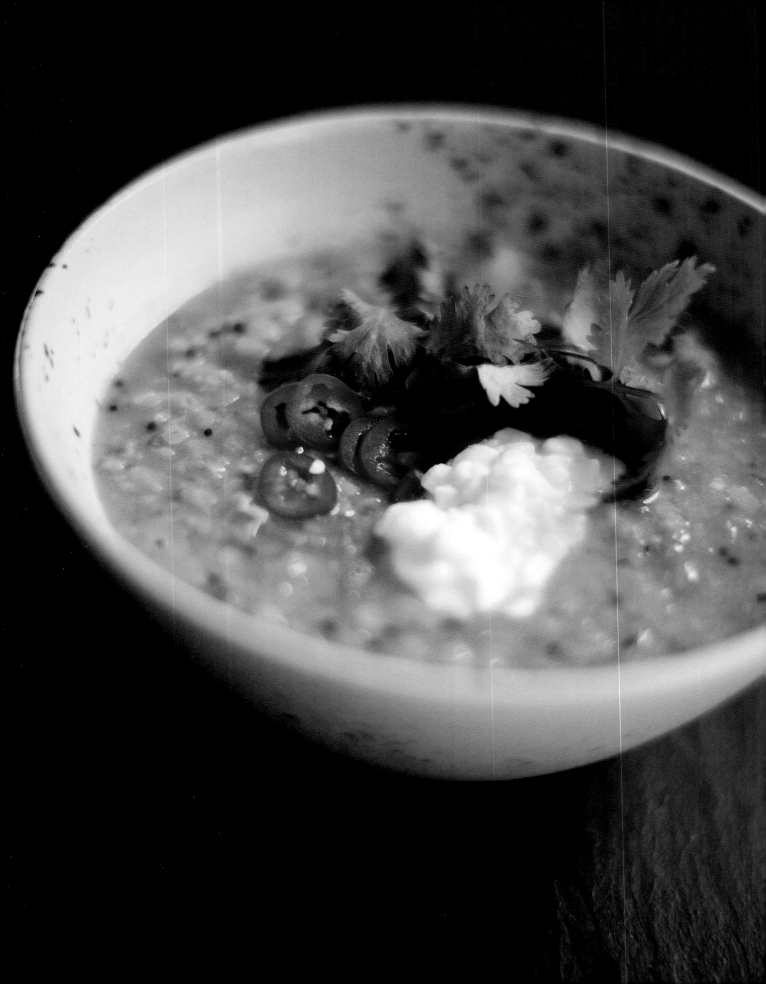

Ginger and Turmeric Dal with Chilies and Cottage Cheese

Peel and mince the onions, ginger, garlic and chili pepper. Rinse and chop the tomatoes into small dices. In a strainer under cold running water, rinse the lentils. Pick through them and remove any stones or blemished lentils. Heat up the oil in a saucepan over low heat and sauté the onions, ginger, garlic, chili pepper and spices until the onions are translucent.

In a medium-sized pot, bring the water to a boil and whisk in the lentils. Turn the heat down to medium-low and cook the lentils for about 25 minutes until they are mushy and tender. Add the tomatoes and onion mixture, then season with salt, pepper, lemon zest and juice to taste. Serve in bowls topped with cottage cheese, chili and fresh coriander.

3 onions

25 g ginger

3 cloves garlic

1 chili pepper

2 large tomatoes

300 g red lentils

30 mL olive oil

1 tsp. ground cumin

1 tsp. mustard seed

1 tsp. ground turmeric

1 tsp. ground paprika

600 mL water

200 g cottage cheese, divided

Salt and pepper, to taste

Zest and juice of 1 lemon

Fresh coriander or cilantro leaves, to serve

Roasted Butternut Squash with Pears and Fresh Basil

Preheat the oven to 175°C/345°F. Line a baking sheet with parchment paper. Halve the butternut squash lengthwise and discard the seeds. Place the butternut squash halves face up on the prepared sheet. Drizzle them with oil, then season with salt and pepper to taste. Roast for about 40–45 minutes until the butternut squash is golden and tender. Remove the pan from the oven and set it aside to cool slightly.

—

Rinse and quarter the pears, cut out the cores, and discard them. Slice the pears into wedges, and marinate them in lime zest and juice. Discard the squash's rind and slice the flesh into wedges. Slice the basil. Plate the butternut squash and pears topped with the basil, salt, pepper and a drizzle of olive oil.

1 medium butternut squash

50 mL olive oil + more for drizzling

3 medium pears

Zest and juice of 1 lime

10 fresh basil leaves

Salt and pepper, to taste

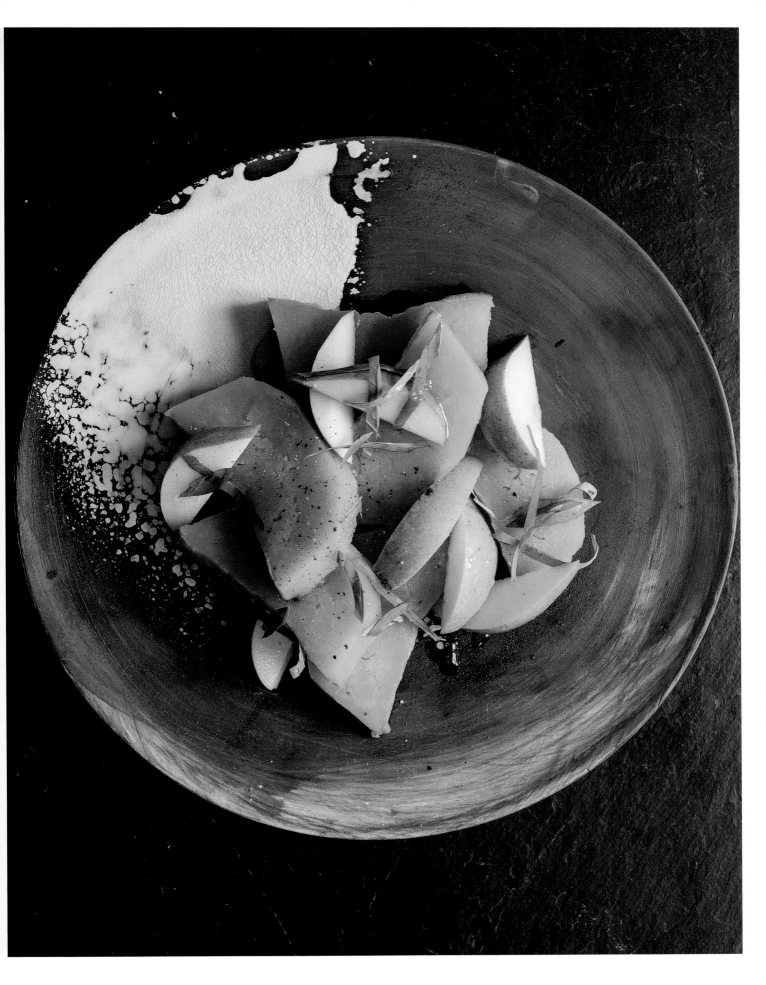

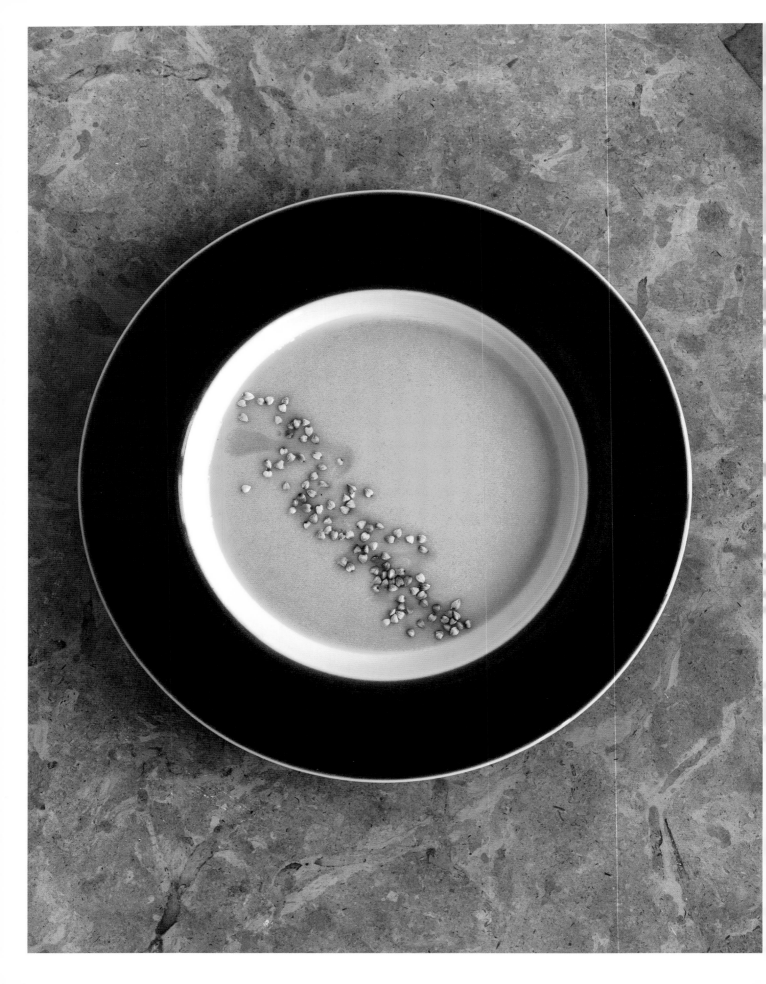

Carrot Ginger Soup with Toasted Buckwheat

Peel the carrots, onions, ginger and garlic, then slice them all thinly. In a large pot, warm up the oil and sauté them over medium heat for about 5 minutes until the onions are soft and translucent. Add the broth to the pot and bring it to a boil. Reduce the heat to medium-low and simmer for 20-25 minutes until the carrots are tender. Remove the pot from the heat. Blend the soup until completely smooth, then pour the soup back into the pot and return it to medium-low heat until it boils. Remove the pot from the heat again and season with the apple cider vinegar, lime juice, salt, pepper and nutmeg to taste.

———

In a small dry pan over medium heat, toast the buckwheat until it is beautifully golden then remove it from the heat. Serve the soup in a bowl, after sprinkling it with buckwheat, drizzling it with olive oil, and topping it with lime zest.

———

TIP: For a spicier version, add a thinly sliced red chili pepper to the sauté pan in the first step.

3 large carrots

2 medium onions

50 g fresh ginger

3 cloves garlic

4 tbsp. olive oil

1.2 L water or chicken broth

Apple cider vinegar, to taste

Salt and pepper, to taste

Freshly grated nutmeg, to taste

50 g buckwheat

Zest and juice of 1 lime

Lamb Chops with Polenta, Carrots, and Mint

8 medium carrots

100 mL olive oil, divided

20 g pine seeds

1000 mL water

1 tsp. salt

200 g dry polenta

100 g freshly grated Parmesan cheese

12 lamb chops (1 kg)

3 lemons, zest and juice

Salt and pepper, to taste

8-10 mint leafs, finely sliced

Scrub and rinse the carrots. Heat up 2 tbsp. of olive oil in a pan and roast the carrots with a pinch of salt over high heat until tender and darkened. Remove them from the pan and keep them warm. Wipe the pan clean and toast the pine seeds for about 2 minutes over medium heat until golden brown.

—

In a saucepan over medium-high heat, bring the water and salt to a boil. Whisk in the polenta. Reduce the heat to low and cook, stirring constantly for 5 minutes until the polenta is smooth and creamy. Add the Parmesan and stir until well combined. Season the polenta with the salt, pepper, lemon zest and juice to taste. Cover the pan and remove it from the heat.

—

Season the lamb chops with salt and pepper to taste. Wipe the pan used for the pine seeds clean. Place it over medium-high heat and warm 1 tbsp. of olive oil. Fry the lamb for 1-2 minutes on each side until red juices come to the surface. Place the lamb on a wire rack and let it rest for 5 minutes before slicing it in half and seasoning with salt and pepper. Spoon a large dollop of polenta onto a dinner plate. Arrange the carrots and lamb in the center of the polenta, then sprinkle with the pine seeds and sliced mint.

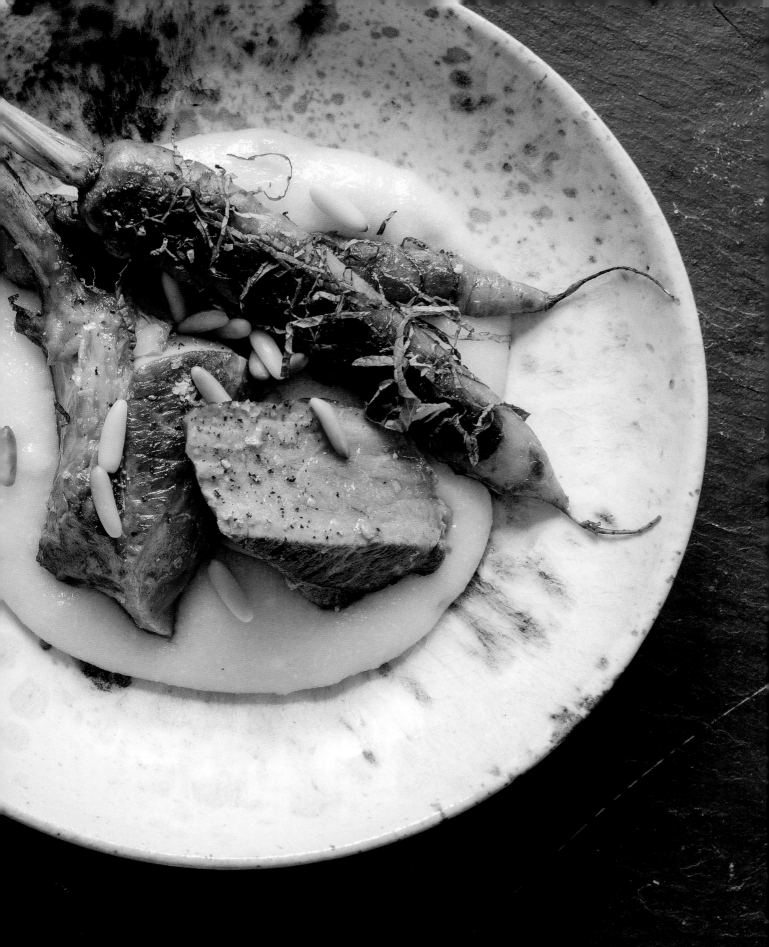

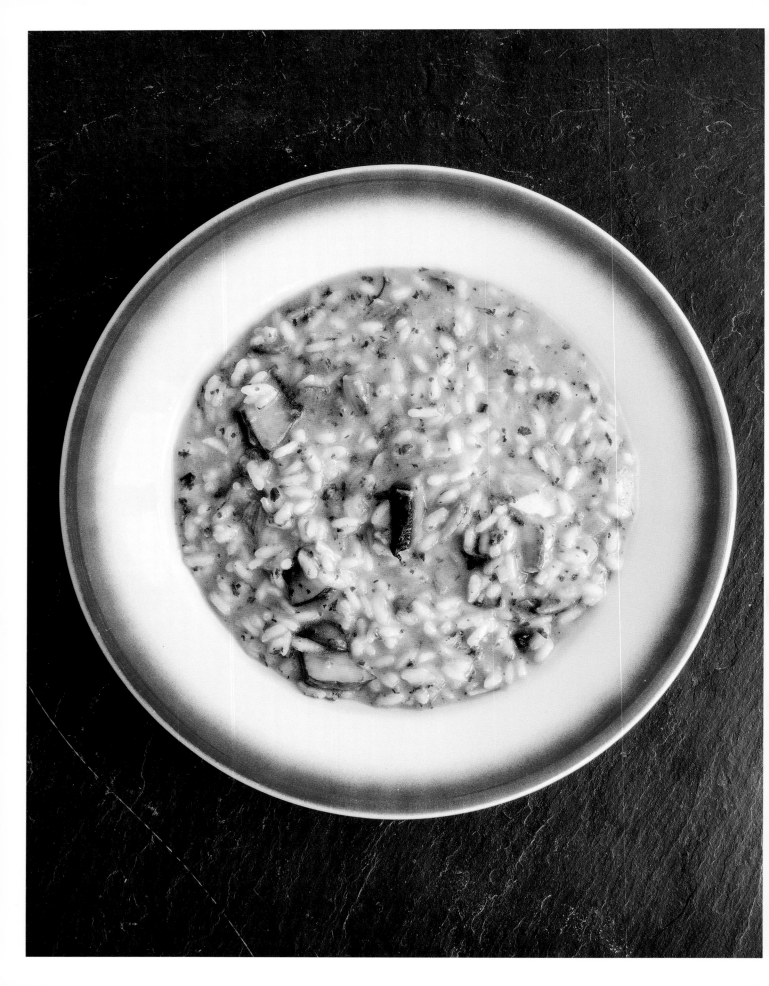

Mushroom Risotto

Clean the mushrooms and slice them. Rinse and pick the thyme and parsley. Blend ½ of the thyme and parsley with 50 mL olive oil until smooth. Peel the onions and garlic, then mince them. Dice the fennel. Warm up 2 tbsp. of olive oil in a cast iron pot, then sauté the onions, garlic and fennel for about 2-3 minutes until the onions are tender and translucent. Add the remaining ½ of the thyme and rice, then stir with a wooden spoon until all the rice grains are coated in oil.

Pour the wine into the rice and cook, stirring constantly until all the liquid has been absorbed. Repeat this process with the water, little by little, until all the liquid has been absorbed into the rice, leaving a creamy fluent risotto. Add the Parmesan to the rice and stir until well combined. Add the mushrooms and parsley purée, then stir until well combined. Season with salt, pepper, lemon zest and juice to taste. Remove the pot from the heat. Serve the risotto in deep plates with additional Parmesan on the side.

6 – 8

500 g mushrooms

1 bunch fresh thyme

½ bunch parsley

2 medium onions

3 cloves garlic

1 medium bulb fennel

500 g risotto rice

250 mL white wine

1250 mL water

50 mL + 4 tbsp. olive oil, divided

200 g freshly grated Parmesan cheese + more to serve

Zest and juice of 1 lemon

Beet and Red Pepper Salad
with Chicken and Ginger Dressing

Rinse and dry the red pepper. Halve it, discard the seeds and white membrane, then slice it thinly. Scrub and mince the ginger finely. Peel the beets and carrots, then shred or julienne them on a Japanese mandolin.

———

Use a stick blender to combine the ginger, lime zest and juice. Add the honey and blend, adding the olive oil little by little. Season with salt and pepper. Toss the beets, carrots, red pepper and chicken with the dressing. Serve in a large salad bowl topped with the fresh coriander and sesame seeds.

1 large red pepper

25 g fresh ginger

400 g raw beets

400 g carrots

Zest and juice of 2 limes

3 tbsp. honey

50 mL olive oil

400 g shredded cooked chicken

Salt and pepper, to taste

1 handful fresh coriander or cilantro

1 tbsp. sesame seeds

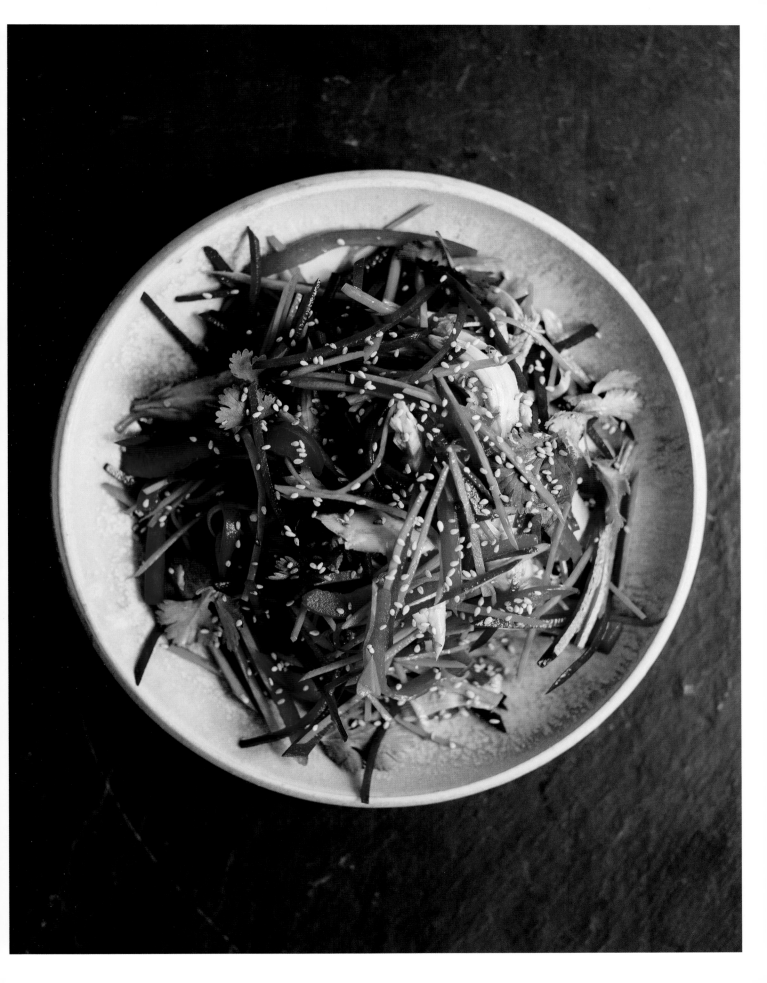

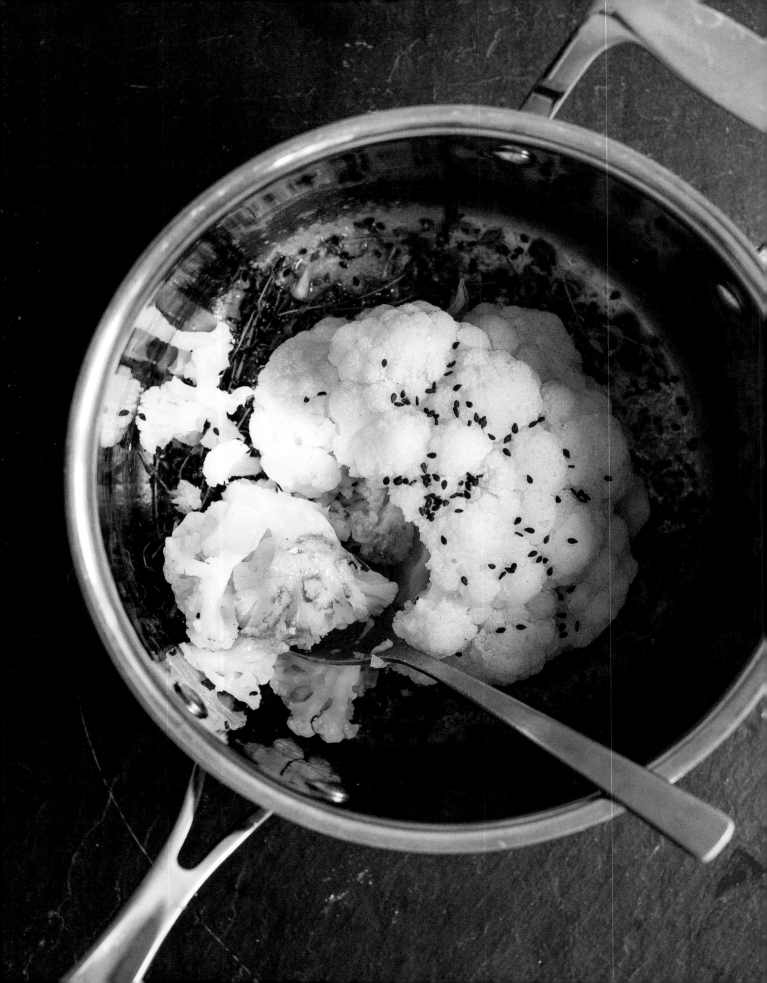

Whole Roasted Cauliflower with Garlic and Nigella Seeds

Rinse the cauliflower. Cut its bottom to create a large flat surface. Rinse the thyme and peel the garlic. In a heavy-bottomed casserole or pot, melt the butter and sprinkle some salt over it. Place the cauliflower in the center, then arrange the thyme and garlic around it. Cover the casserole with a lid and cook over medium-low heat for 25-30 minutes until the cauliflower is tender and its bottom is caramelized. Sprinkle it with salt and the nigella seeds before serving it in the pot.

1 medium head cauliflower

½ bunch fresh thyme

1 head garlic

50 g butter, cubed

10 g nigella or black onion seeds

Salt, to taste

Endive with Beet Purée and Brown Butter

Rinse the beets, cover them with water in a pot, and bring them to a boil over medium heat until completely tender. Put on single-use gloves and squeeze the skin off the beets, then blend them into a fine purée in a food processor or blender. Season with balsamic vinegar and salt to taste.

———

In a saucepan over low heat, melt the butter. Allow the milk solids to caramelize and brown slowly. Whisk occasionally until the butter is golden brown and smells like toasted nuts. Rinse the endive heads and cut them lengthwise into long thin wedges. Plate a handful of the wedges on a large spoonful of beet purée, then top them with a spoonful of browned butter to serve.

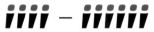

300 g beets

Balsamic vinegar, to taste

Salt, to taste

100 g butter

4 medium heads endive

Flaked salt, to serve

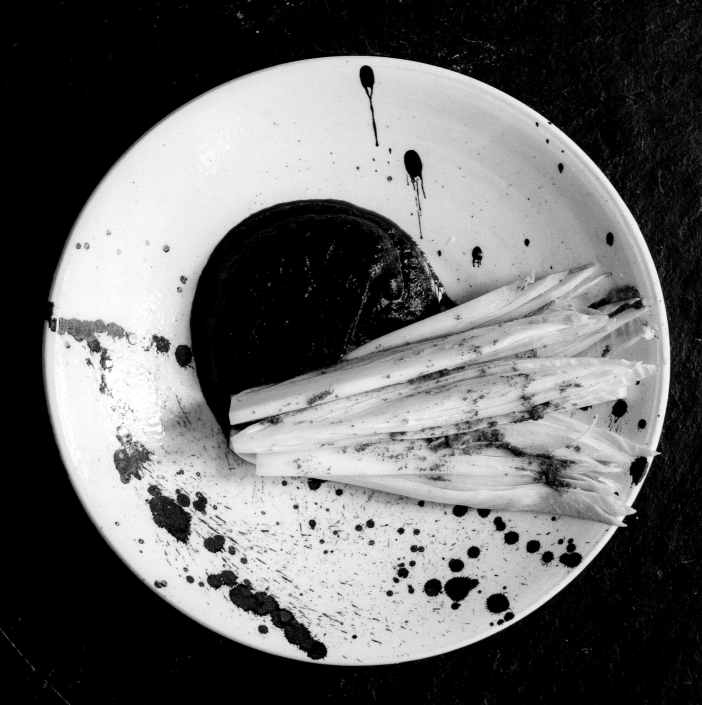

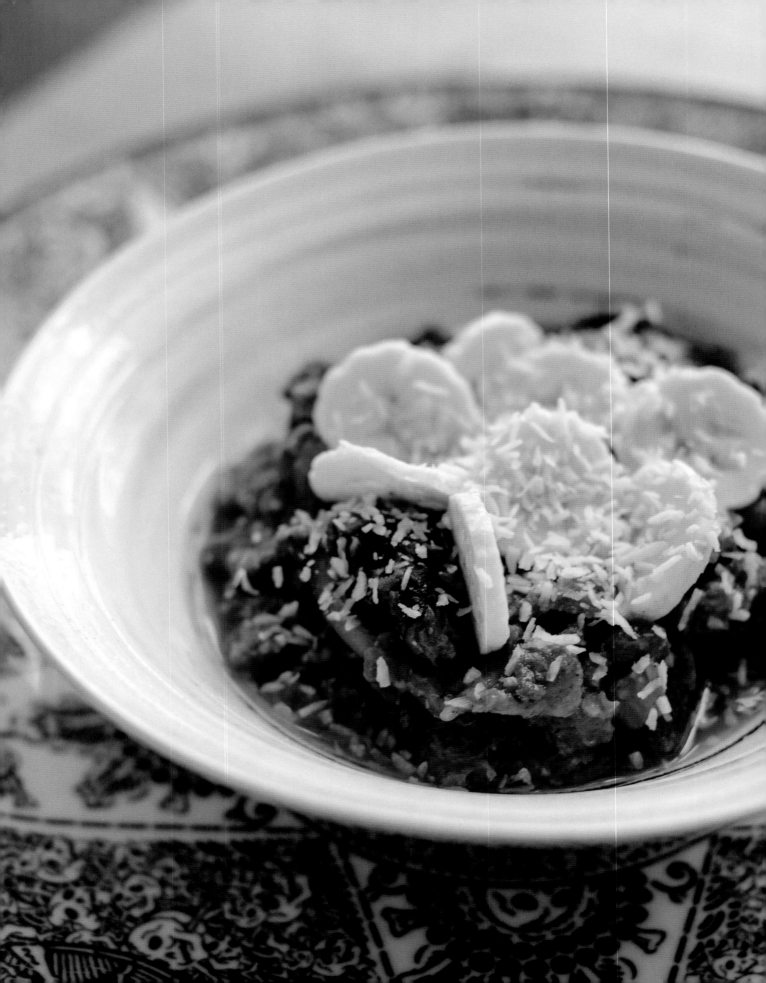

Spiced Veal Stew with Coconut and Banana

G D N

Peel the garlic, scrub the ginger, and mince them. Peel the carrots and onions, then cut them into 0.5 cm-thick slices. Rinse and dice the eggplants into 3 cm x 3 cm cubes, then sprinkle them with salt. In a large mixing bowl, combine the veal, apple cider vinegar, garlic, ginger, garam masala and cloves. Season with salt and pepper, then set it aside to marinate.

———

In a large, deep, heavy-bottomed Dutch oven over medium-high heat, warm the oil and brown the veal for about 3-4 minutes until caramelized. Add the carrots, onions, eggplants and raisins, then sauté for 2 minutes. Add the broth to the pot and bring to a boil. Reduce the heat to medium-low and let it simmer under a lid for 45-50 minutes until the veal is completely tender. Remove the pot from the heat. Season the stew with salt, pepper and balsamic vinegar to taste. Serve with the steamed rice topped with sliced bananas and shredded coconut.

3 cloves garlic

50 g fresh ginger

2 medium carrots

2 medium onions

2 medium eggplants

400 g veal rump, diced

50 mL apple cider vinegar

2 tbsp. garam masala

1 pinch crushed cloves

4 tbsp. olive oil

20 g raisins

500 mL water or broth

2 medium bananas, peeled and sliced

20 g shredded coconut

Steamed rice, to serve

Shaved Brussels Sprout Salad with Blackberries and Cottage Cheese

Peel and slice the onions thinly, then soak the slices in cold water as you prepare the remaining ingredients. Rinse the Brussels sprouts. Trim off the bottom ends and discard any damaged outer leaves. Shave the Brussels sprouts on a Japanese mandolin directly into a serving bowl. Rinse, pick and slice the parsley. Rinse and slice the blackberries in half. Add the onions, cottage cheese and parsley to the serving bowl, then toss lightly.

⸻

In a small mixing bowl, combine the lime zest and juice. Stir in the honey. While whisking constantly, drizzle in the olive oil. Season with salt and pepper to taste. Toss the salad with half of the blackberries and vinaigrette. Serve it topped with the remaining blackberries.

1 medium white onion

500 g Brussels sprouts

1 bunch fresh flat-leaf parsley

50 g fresh blackberries, rinsed and dried

Zest and juice of 2 limes

100 g cottage cheese

2 tbsp. honey

50 mL olive oil

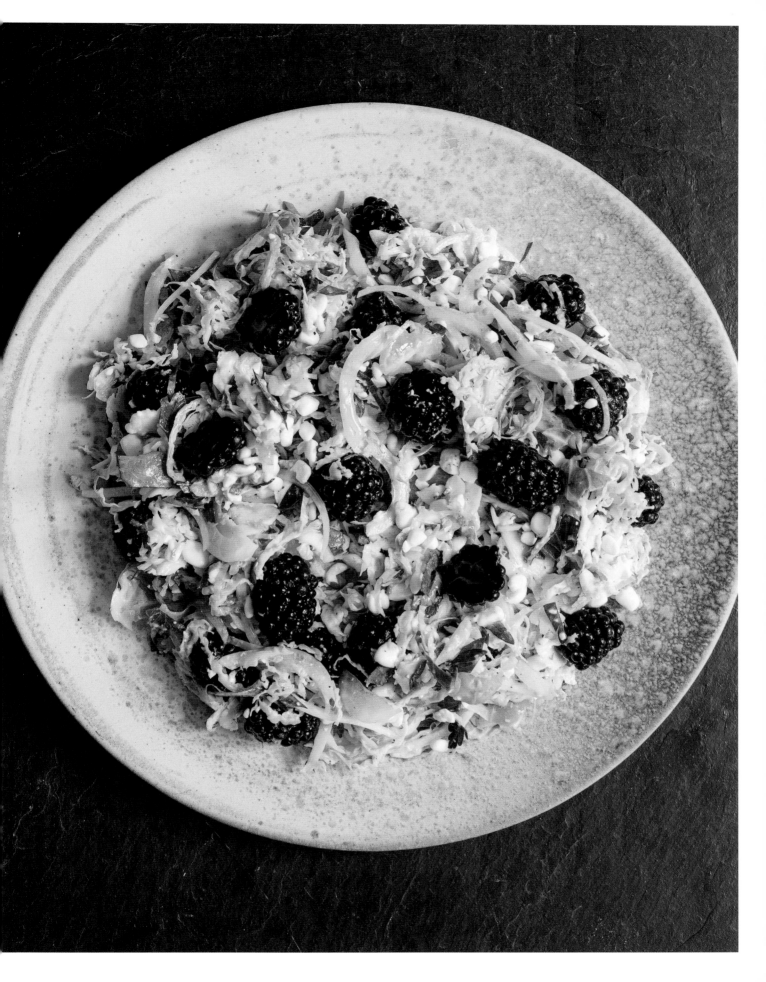

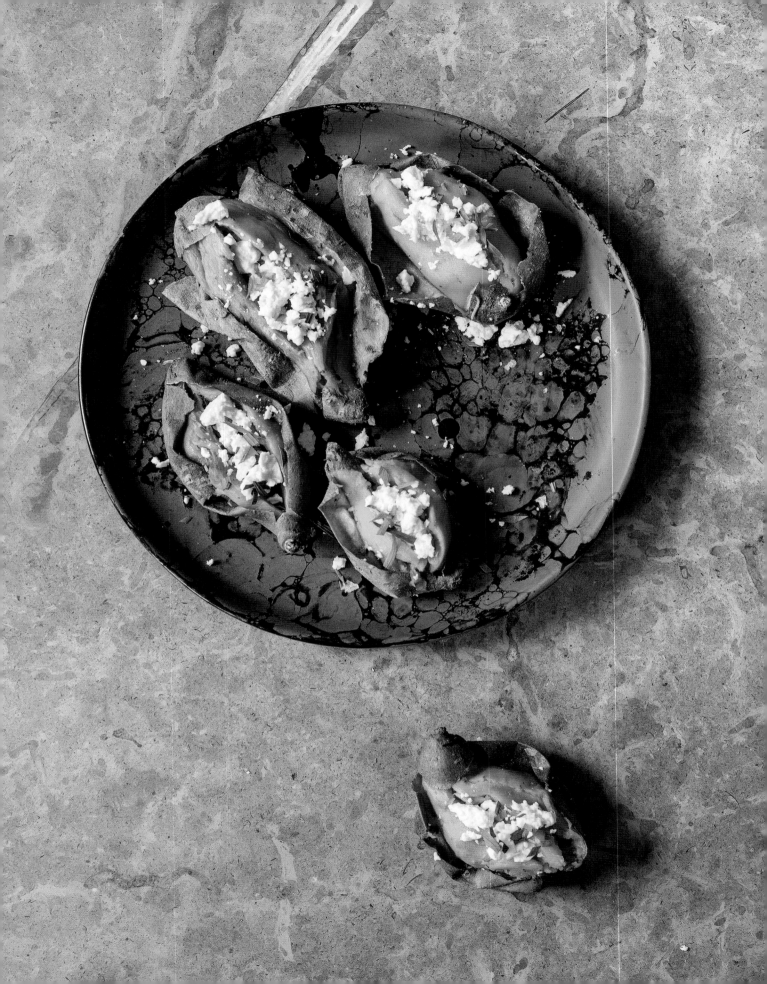

Sweet Potatoes with Goat Cheese and Tarragon

Preheat the oven to 160°C/320°F. Line a baking sheet with parchment paper. Wash the potatoes and place them onto the prepared sheet. Bake for 35– 40 minutes until they are completely tender. Remove them from the oven and set them aside to cool.

Using a sharp knife, make a long incision in each sweet potato and push the sides open. Plate the sweet potatoes on a serving platter, then top them with crumbled fresh cheese and tarragon. Add the lime zest, juice and a drizzle of olive oil, then serve.

600 g sweet potatoes

50 g fresh cheese, crumbled

3 sprigs fresh tarragon, stemmed

Zest and juice of 1 lime

3 tbsp. olive oil

Salt and pepper, to taste

Breads, Cakes and Desserts

"Performance and recovery are both heavily influenced by the food you eat.
The wrong foods before a competition can wreck your day in a hurry."

SELENE YEAGER

Born — 21 Feburary 1969
Professional since — 2010
Origin — U.S.A.
Lives in — Pennsylvania

Selene Yeager - Fit Chick, health journalist, author, athlete and coach - started fantasizing about steak on long rides after her daughter was born. However, she also knows exactly how important the right diet is for an endurance athlete. "It's essential for day-to-day performance and recovery, as well as keeping healthy and energetic," she says. "Performance and recovery are both heavily influenced by the food you eat. The wrong foods before a competition can wreck your day in a hurry."

Selene says she doesn't follow a certain diet per se, but tries to eat fresh, unprocessed foods when possible. "When you travel for events a lot, I believe you also need to be trained to be flexible so you're not freaking out when your plane gets in late, you're out of your special rolled oats, and all you have is some Taco Bell somewhere!" She believes that if you're smart about your nutrition, you can get good food that works for you nearly anywhere. So what works for her? "I do best with mostly vegetables, lean protein and fat with a portion of complex carbs in the form of grains," she tells me. Has she ever cut out sugar or gone low-carb? "When I try to cut grains out, I end up trolling the kitchen eating a bunch of chocolates and other sweets! If I try to do the very low-carb thing, sh*t goes sideways."

The night before an event, Selene eats steak, salad and some grains, then oats, nut butter and Greek yogurt for breakfast. She doesn't eat much just before the race - "just a bite of a bar, perhaps" - and what she eats during the race depends on the duration of the event: chews and gels over a shorter time, or figs, dates and fig/date bars when she's facing a tougher course. Whatever the distance, she recovers immediately afterwards with a protein drink and treats herself to a beer, a glass of wine, "or whatever I want" in the evening.

Selene eats a wide variety of food, but a typical day entails eggs and vegetables in the morning, some protein and vegetables for lunch, and some protein, carbs and vegetables for dinner. She also indulges in dark chocolate and "too much coffee" daily. The way food looks and tastes are super important to her, especially when she loses her appetite after a long day of training or competing: "It can last for a few hours or even into the next day. However, my appetite usually comes roaring back after my recovery spin." The more attractive and palatable food is, she adds, the more it helps her to refuel. I wonder aloud if an athlete needs to think about other factors like heat and the cold, and she agrees with me completely. "Absolutely! I can eat a pizza out there and be fine when it's cold. Heat messes with me, and I have to eat more carefully."

With the rising popularity of vegan and vegetarian diets, I ask Selene if she'd consider them. She divulges that she used to be a vegetarian for 10 years, and acknowledges that those diets are "great if they work for you, but I'd only consider going back to being a vegetarian if someone cooked for me." Her favorite plate on- and off-season is still a good piece of steak and a big pile of fresh greens.

Selene is definitely doing something right. In her first ever Ironman event in Kentucky U.S.A., she emerged victorious in her age group before making it all the way to the Ironman World Championships. Besides her focus on nutrition, she alternates her workouts with a couple of hard days, a couple of moderate days, an easy day, and one very long day. She supplements her endurance training with CrossFit twice a week, and a session of hot yoga.

When asked if she has any specific advice for women athletes, she tells me that hydration is key, as are carbs and protein. "I think women have less margins for error because of our limited muscle mass and the impact of hormonal fluctuations." What about new triathletes who want to eat right, be full of energy, and even lose weight? "Don't get caught up in what everyone else is doing," she cautions. "Find what works for you. People are not test tubes. There are a million different ways to eat, because not one singular way works for everyone."

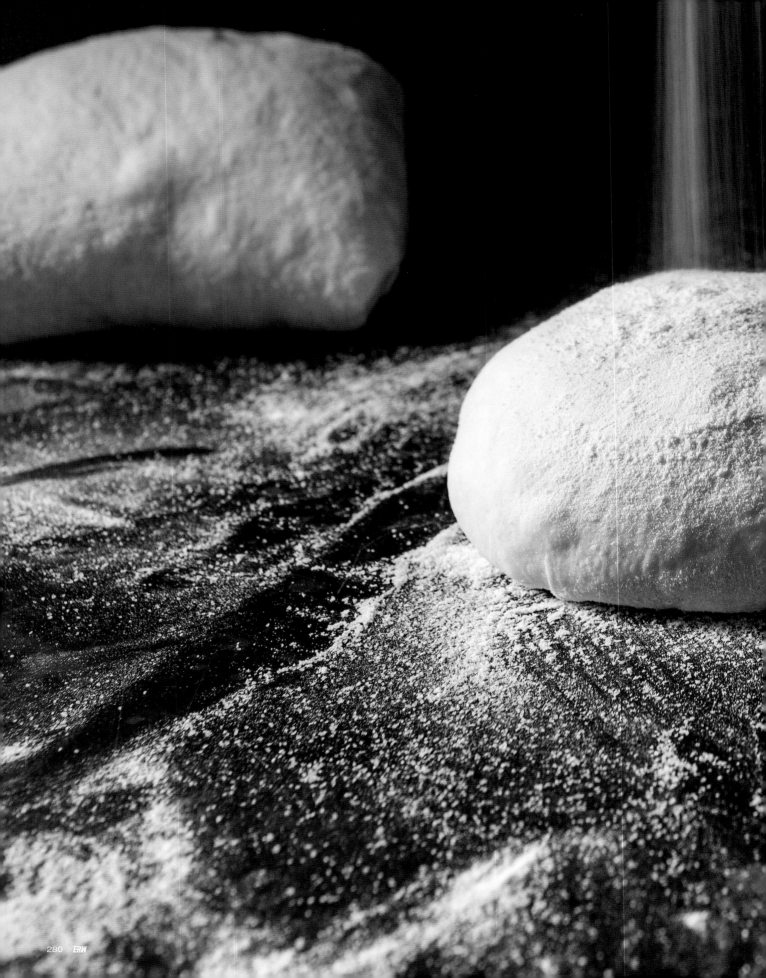

Wheat Bread

I do not use much wheat anymore, but when I do, I make bread - really good sourdough bread. Unfortunately, there is no way to make it without investing significant time in the process, since the flavor must develop gradually as the dough ferments.

My Sourdough Bread recipe is a great basic wheat bread recipe, where you can add your own twists with seeds, nuts, dried fruit and spices to change it up to your liking. If you do end up making a habit of baking bread often, I recommend that you keep my Basic Sourdough Starter (see recipe on p.284) going in the refrigerator. Besides adding much more flavor to the result, you will eventually be able to leave yeast out of your recipes entirely.

Hannah's Sourdough Bread

Day 1 preparations:

In a small mixing bowl, dissolve the sourdough starter and yeast in the water. Transfer the mixture into the bowl of a stand mixer fitted with the kneading attachment, or a large mixing bowl. Add the flour and salt and knead, either with your hands or on low speed if using the stand mixer, for 5 minutes. Cover it with plastic wrap and set it aside for 30 minutes at room temperature.

Knead again until the dough is smooth and elastic. Cover it and set it aside at room temperature again for about 1 hour, until the dough doubles in size. Knead again, cover it with plastic wrap, and refrigerate overnight. Remember, the dough will rise, so ensure that the mixing bowl is large enough to accommodate the much larger dough.

Day 2 preparations:

Preheat the oven to 250°C/480°F. If you are baking in loaf pans – grease 4 silicone loaf pans. If you are shaping rolls or baguettes and baking on a baking sheet – line a baking sheet with parchment paper. Dust a clean, flat work surface with about ½ of the rice flour and carefully turn out the dough onto the surface without puncturing it. (If the dough is too soft to work with, quarter it using a dough cutter or knife and transfer it onto the loaf pans immediately to bake as loaves.)

Fold the dough like an envelope: Firstly, fold from the work surface's edges up towards the center. Next, fold the sides in, then lastly, fold up toward the last open part, making one large piece of dough. If you are baking in loaf pans – using a dough cutter or knife, quarter the dough and transfer each piece onto a prepared pan. Cover it with plastic wrap and set it aside to rise to room temperature. If you are shaping rolls or baguettes and baking on a baking sheet – carefully roll the dough into a thickness of 5 cm. Using a dough cutter or knife, divide the dough into 16–20 rolls or 2–3 baguettes. Transfer the rolls or baguettes onto the baking sheet. Dust with the remaining rice flour. Using a kitchen towel, cover them and set them aside to rise to room temperature. Using a razor blade or a very sharp knife, score the surface of the rolls or baguettes into your desired pattern.

To bake the bread:

Speed and efficiency are key! With a cup of warm water at hand, open the oven door and quickly move the loaf pans or baking sheet to the middle of the oven. Pour the warm water into the bottom of the oven and quickly close the door. The water will evaporate and steam the bread, making the crust thin and crispy. Reduce the oven temperature to 220°C/425°F and bake for another 15 –20 minutes, depending on the size of your loaves, rolls, or baguettes. The bread is ready when it is golden and makes a hollow sound when you tap it. Remove it from the oven and set it aside on a wire rack to cool before slicing.

When the bread has cooled completely, carefully wrap the loaves, rolls, or baguettes you will not eat over the following days with plastic wrap and store them in the freezer. Plastic-wrapped bread can easily be re-baked when needed for that straight-out-of-the-oven bread sensation.

——

To re-bake frozen bread: Preheat the oven to 200°C/395°F. Defrost and unwrap the bread. Run it quickly under the tap to wet its surface without letting it soak up too much water, or its crust will be too hard. Place the bread directly onto the oven rack and bake for 5-7 minutes until the crust is crispy and the bread is warmed through.

Yield: 16-20 rolls / ~3-4 loaves

100 g basic sourdough starter (see recipe on p.284)

5 g dry or 10 g fresh yeast

700 mL water, divided

1 kg wheat flour

20 g salt

50 g rice flour, to dust

100 mL warm water, to bake

Basic Sourdough Starter

To prepare the sourdough starter: In a mixing bowl, stir the water and flour together. Cover it with plastic wrap and set it aside at room temperature overnight.

To use the sourdough starter: Your sourdough starter is ready when it bubbles and smells sour. To keep it going, you will need to 'feed' it, which means that once you have used a part of it to make your bread dough, you will need to mix in a new batch of sourdough starter into the existing one and place the new mixture directly into the refrigerator. Keep it refrigerated between baking sessions.

TIP: If you do not 'feed' your sourdough starter often enough, it will over-ferment and you will need to start over. Tend to it and check it daily. If you keep it going, it will reward you with the tastiest bread you can imagine.

100 g all-purpose or whole-wheat flour

100 mL water

Nut and Seed Bread

Ⓖ Ⓓ Ⓥ

Preheat the oven to 150°C/300°F. Grease 1 silicone loaf pan. In a large mixing bowl, combine the mixed seeds, nuts and chia seeds. In a separate mixing bowl, whisk the eggs, olive oil, vinegar and salt together. Combine the 2 mixtures well. Pour the batter into the prepared loaf pan. Bake for 35-40 minutes, depending on the height of your loaf. The bread is ready when it is completely firm and golden. Remove it from the oven and set it aside on a wire rack to cool completely before slicing. For a longer shelf life, wrap it well with plastic wrap and refrigerate it for up to 1 week.

TIP: This recipe is quite versatile. For variations, maintain the 600 g measure for your dry ingredients but try:
- Substituting ⅙ of the nuts and seeds with dried fruits
- Adding spices and coconut
- Adding shredded carrots or beets

Yield: 1 loaf

600 g mixed seeds and nuts (sunflower seeds, flax seeds, pumkin seeds etc.)

1 tbsp. chia seeds

6 whole large eggs

2 tbsp. olive oil

1 tbsp. apple cider vinegar

1 tsp. salt

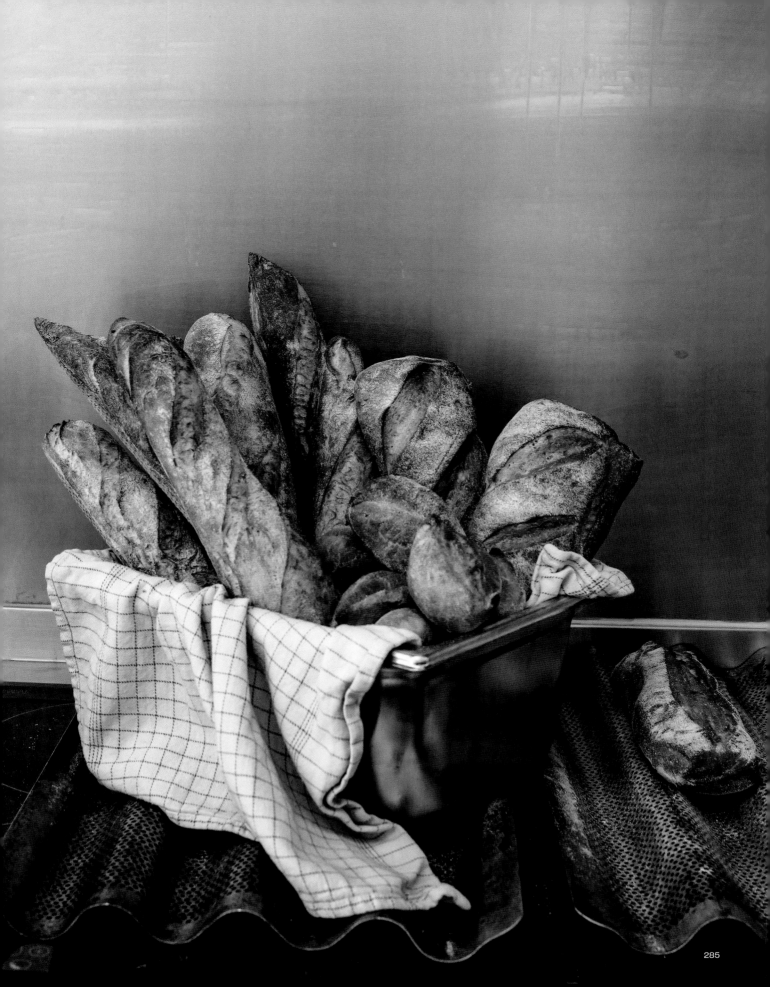

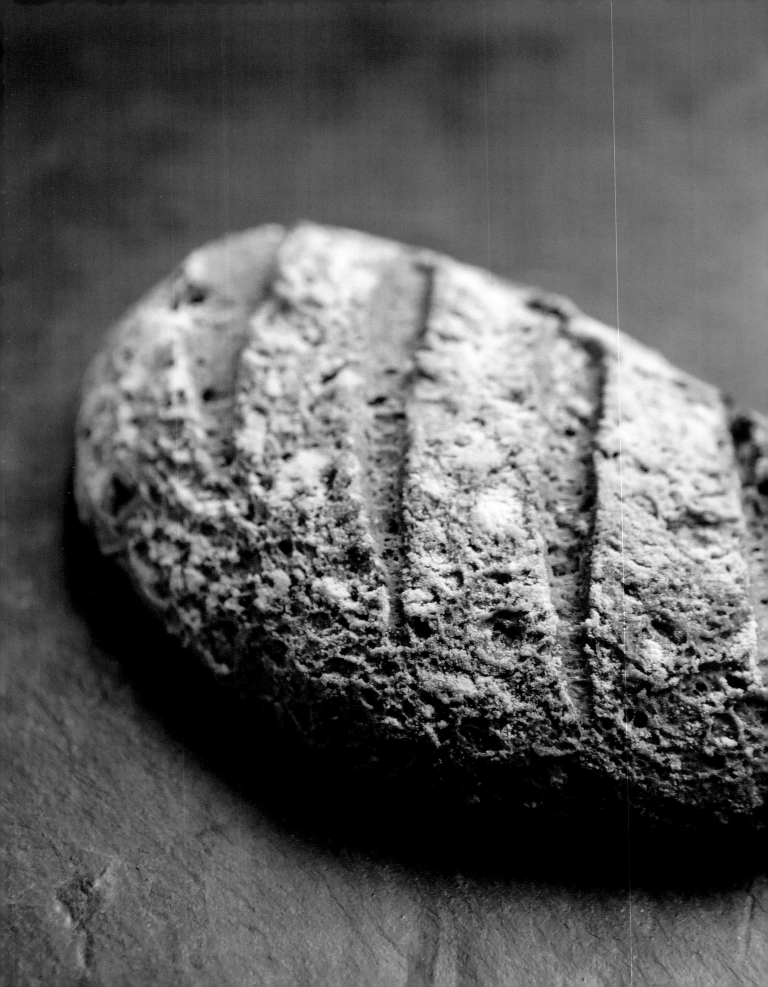

Wheat- and Gluten-free Brown Loaf

G D N V

Day 1 preparations:

In a large mixing bowl, sift the potato starch, rice flour, sorghum flour, psyllium, apple cider vinegar, yeast, baking powder, salt and sugar together. Add the egg, 3 tbsp. olive oil and water, then knead together until smooth. Grease a very large bowl with the remaining 1 tbsp. of oil and transfer the dough to it. Cover it with plastic wrap and refrigerate overnight.

Day 2 preparations:

Preheat the oven to 200°C/395°F. Line a baking sheet with parchment paper. Dust a clean, flat work surface with the rice flour and turn out the dough onto the surface. Using a dough cutter or knife, halve the dough and transfer each piece to the prepared baking sheet. Using a razor blade or a very sharp knife and score the surface of the rolls or baguettes into your desired pattern. Cover them with a kitchen towel and set them aside to rise to room temperature. Bake for 25-30 minutes until golden. The bread is ready when it is golden brown and makes a hollow sound when you tap it. Remove it from the oven and set it aside on a wire rack to cool completely before slicing.

TIP: Store uneaten bread in a plastic bag at room temperature for a longer shelf life.

Yield: 2 loaves

200 g potato starch

180 g rice flour

120 g sorghum flour

1 tbsp. psyllium husk

1 tbsp. apple cider vinegar

1 tbsp. active dry yeast

1 tbsp. baking powder

1 tsp. fine salt

1 tsp. sugar

1 whole large egg

3 tbsp. olive oil + 1 tbsp. olive oil, to grease

500 mL warm water

25 g rice flour, to dust

"One Dough Fits All"

Version 1: Use the dough straight away

Version 2: Knead the dough together again and refrigerate in a covered bowl overnight for flavor, texture and more air to develop.

This is the most amazing bread dough ever, whichever version you choose! With this simple recipe, you can create rolls, loaves, flatbreads, pita breads, pizza crusts, baguettes and anything your bready heart desires. I use brown rice flour to shape my dough, as it does not burn as fast and gives my bread a nice crunch, but you can use semolina or regular flour as substitutes.

Combine the water and yeast. Mix in the flour and salt, then knead by hand or in an electrical mixer until smooth. Cover the mixing bowl with plastic wrap and let the dough rise at room temperature until its size doubles.

———

TIP: I always save a small handful of dough in an airtight container in the fridge for my next baking session, as this adds natural flavor and fermentation to the dough.

800 mL water

2 g dry yeast

1000 g wheat flour

15 g salt

100 g left-over sour dough (optional)

Bread and Rolls

Ⓓ Ⓝ Ⓥ

Preheat the oven to 220°C/425°F. Dust a clean work surface with flour and carefully place the dough onto the table without puncturing it too much. Fold the dough in 3, by folding 2 sides into the middle. Repeat on the long side afterwards. For bread - divide the dough into 2 or 4 loafs. For rolls - cut the dough into 12-16 rolls.

———

Place the dough onto a rice flour-dusted baking tin lined with parchment paper. Bake the bread for 25-30 minutes or the rolls for 15-18 minutes until golden brown. The bread should make a hollow sound when you tap it. For both options, set aside to cool down before cutting for the best results.

Yield: 2-4 loaves / 12-16 rolls

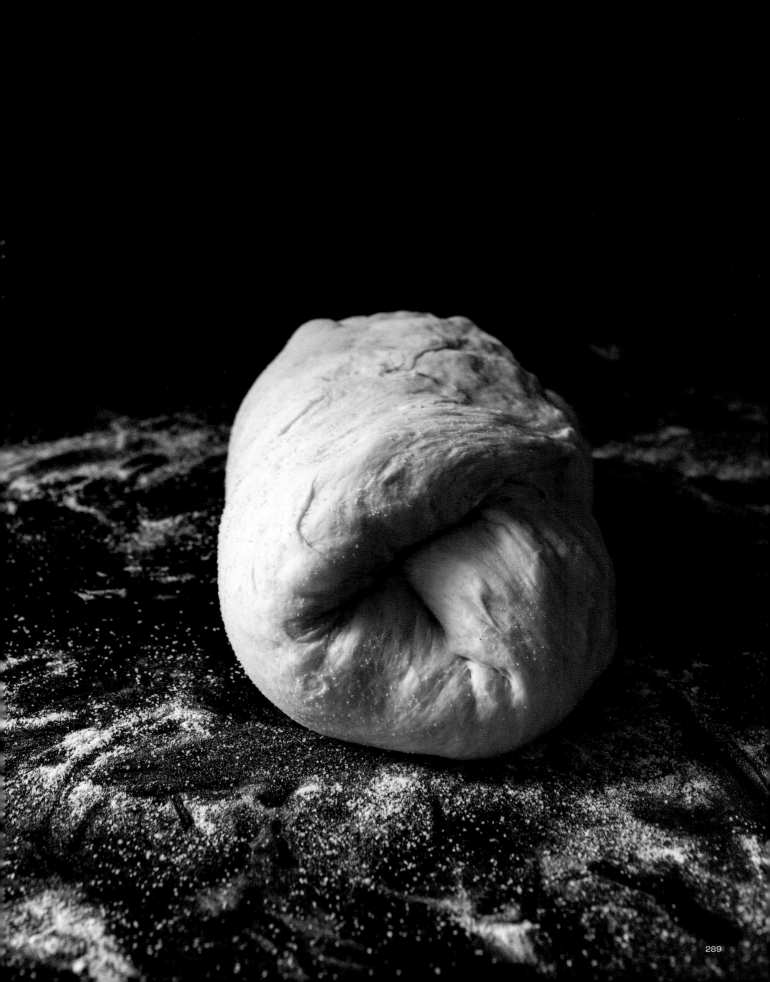

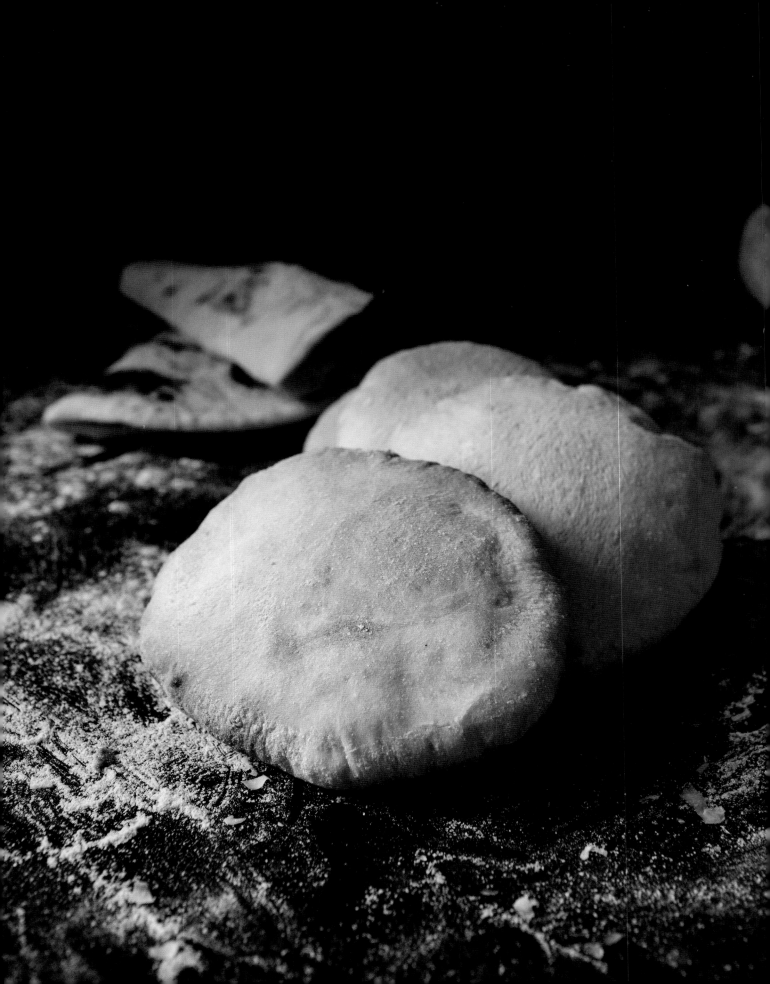

Flatbread

Use dough version 1.

Divide the dough into 20 even pieces and roll them into little balls. Dust a clean work surface with flour and roll each ball as thinly as possible with a rolling pin or a glass bottle with no label on it. Heat up a pan over high heat and add 1 tsp. of olive oil. Sprinkle a pinch of salt onto the pan and fry the flat dough for about 1 minute on each side until it puffs up. The bread should have spots of dark color for the best flavor. Stack and eat straight away, store in an airtight container for 3 days, or freeze to be reheated.

Pita Bread

Use dough version 1 or 2.

Preheat the oven to 300°C/575°F (or as high as possible) with a pizza stone or a cast iron pan inside. Divide the dough into 20 even pieces and roll them into little balls. Dust a clean work surface with flour, and roll each ball flat (1-2 mm) with a rolling pin or a glass bottle with no label on it. Line the pizza stone with parchment paper. Place 1 pita dough onto the pizza stone at a time, and bake for 2-3 minutes until it is fully puffed up and light golden. Flip it over and bake for another 30 seconds. Remove it and let it cool down slightly before serving.

Pizza Makes 4-6

Use dough version 2 for the best results.

———

Preheat the oven to 300°C/575°F with a pizza stone or a metal baking tray placed upside down inside. Knead the dough until smooth, divide it into 4 or 6 portions and roll them out as thinly as possible. Transfer them onto a piece of parchment paper, then spread 50 g of tomato sauce and add cheese onto each pizza dough. Slide the dough onto the hot tray and bake for 10-12 minutes until the dough is crisp and golden brown. Carefully slide the pizza onto a wire rack and top it with sliced ham, rocket salad and garlic oil. Prebake pizza bottoms with tomato sauce and let them cool down on a wire rack. Freeze them for later use and add toppings to your liking.

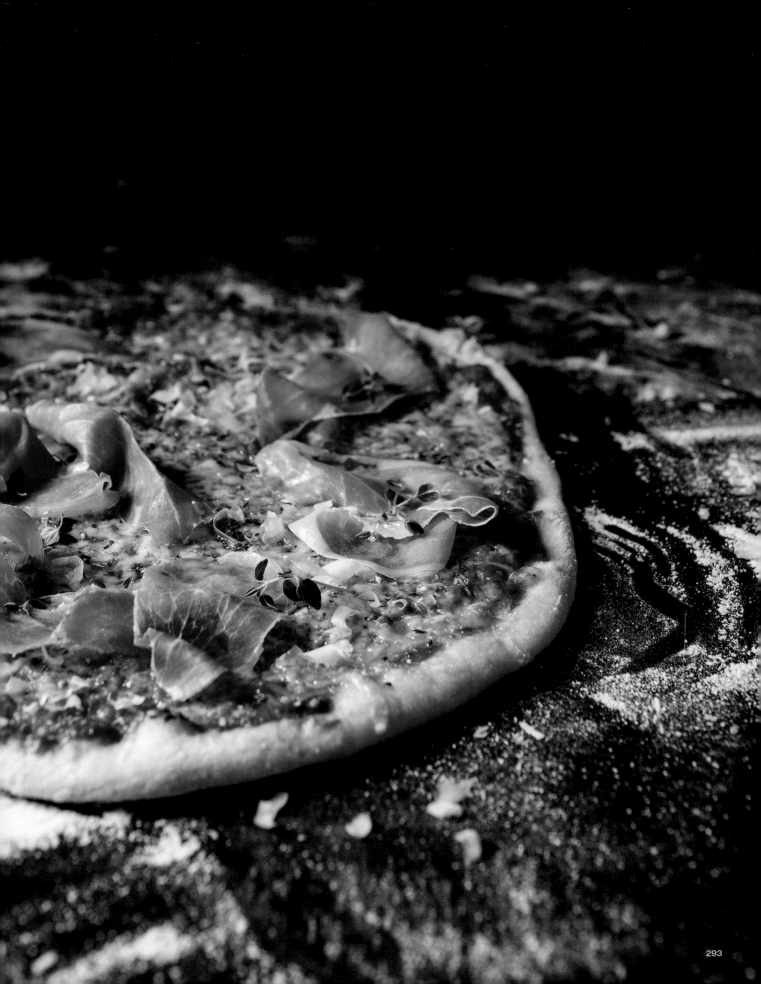

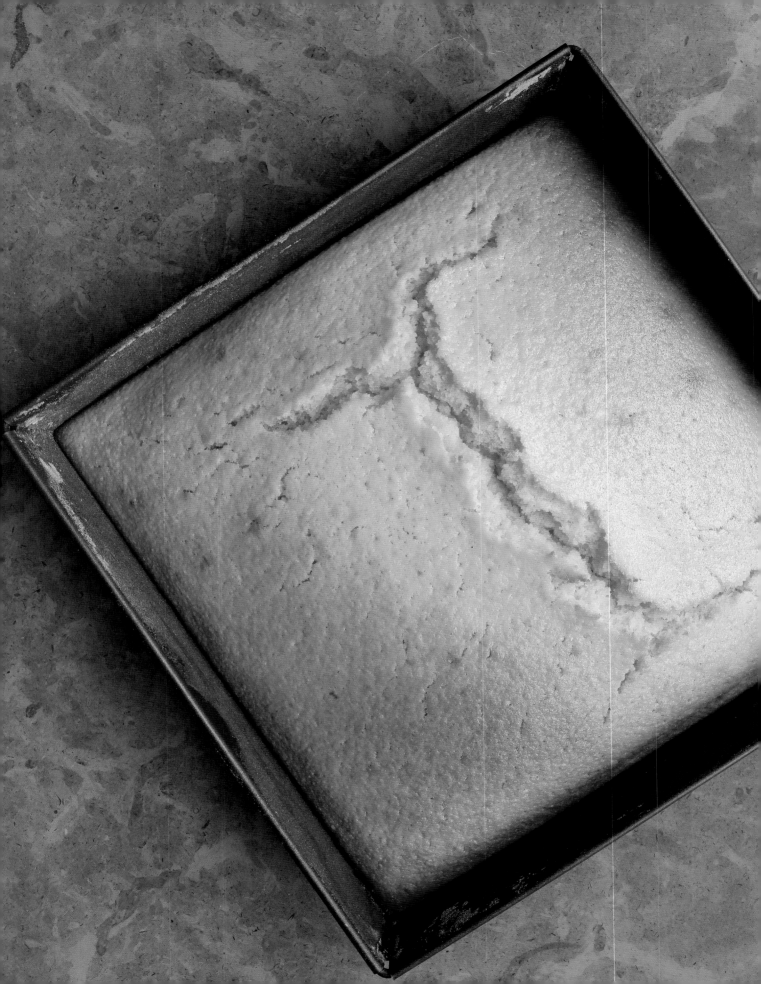

Basic Wheat-free Cake

G D V

Preheat the oven to 150°C/300°F. Grease 1 cake pan or 2 silicone loaf pans. In a mixing bowl, sift together the rice flour, ground cinnamon, baking powder, salt, and xanthan gum. Mix in the nuts, sugar and cornmeal. In a separate large mixing bowl, whisk the eggs and oil together. Blend the dry ingredients gradually into the wet ingredients. Fold in ⅔ of the diced fruit mixture.

Transfer the batter into the prepared cake pan or loaf pans. Bake for 35–40 minutes, until a cake tester or toothpick inserted into the center comes out clean. The cake is ready when it is firm and golden. Remove it from the oven and set it aside on a wire rack to cool completely before slicing and serving.

TIP: I love basic recipes! With this one, you can create your own combinations depending on the season and mood. Instead of wheat flour, feel free to make your own favorite flour mixture. For variations, why not try these yummy combinations below?
- Peaches, almonds, and white chocolate
- Apples, fresh thyme, and hazelnuts
- Rhubarb, coconut, pears, pecans, and dark chocolate
- Plums, pistachios, and cardamom

Yield: 2 loaves

150 g rice flour

1 tsp. ground cinnamon

1 tsp. baking powder

½ tsp. fine salt

½ tsp. xanthan gum

65 g chopped nuts, shredded coconut or chocolate chips

250 g granulated sugar

150 g cornmeal

4 whole large eggs

175 mL vegetable oil

6 medium fresh fruits (apples, plums, peaches, nectarines, etc.) diced into 1cm cubes

Basic Frozen Banana Ice Cream

Ⓖ Ⓝ Ⓥ

In the bowl of a food processor fitted with the S-blade attachment, then process the bananas until well puréed. Add the yogurt and vanilla seeds, then season with lemon zest and juice to taste. Serve immediately or freeze in an airtight container for later.

—

TIP: This recipe works brilliantly with brown or over-ripe bananas, as they are much sweeter. Peel and freeze them beforehand.
For variations, you can easily change up the flavors by blending in other frozen berries and fruits or folding chocolate chips, nuts and other flavors into the mixture after it has been blended.

Ideas for combinations:
- Frozen pineapple and mint
- Mint and chocolate chips
- Peanut butter, orange zest and cocoa powder
- Elderflower or violets
- Dulce de leche

Yield: 2-3 portions

4 peeled frozen bananas

4 tbsp. plain Greek yogurt

½ vanilla bean

Zest and juice of 1 lemon

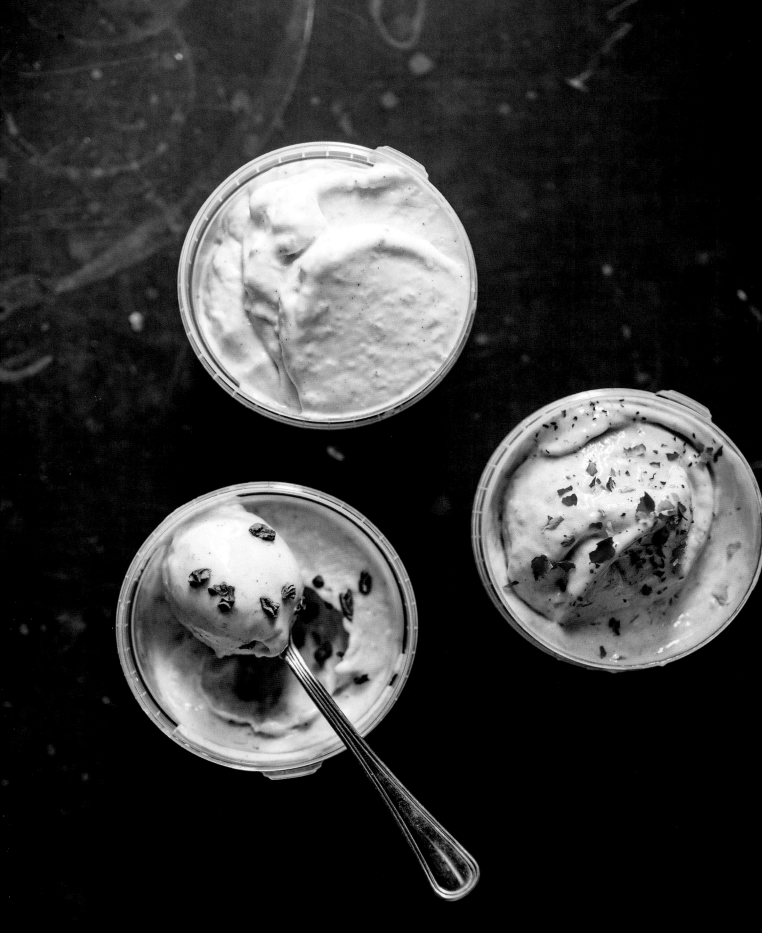

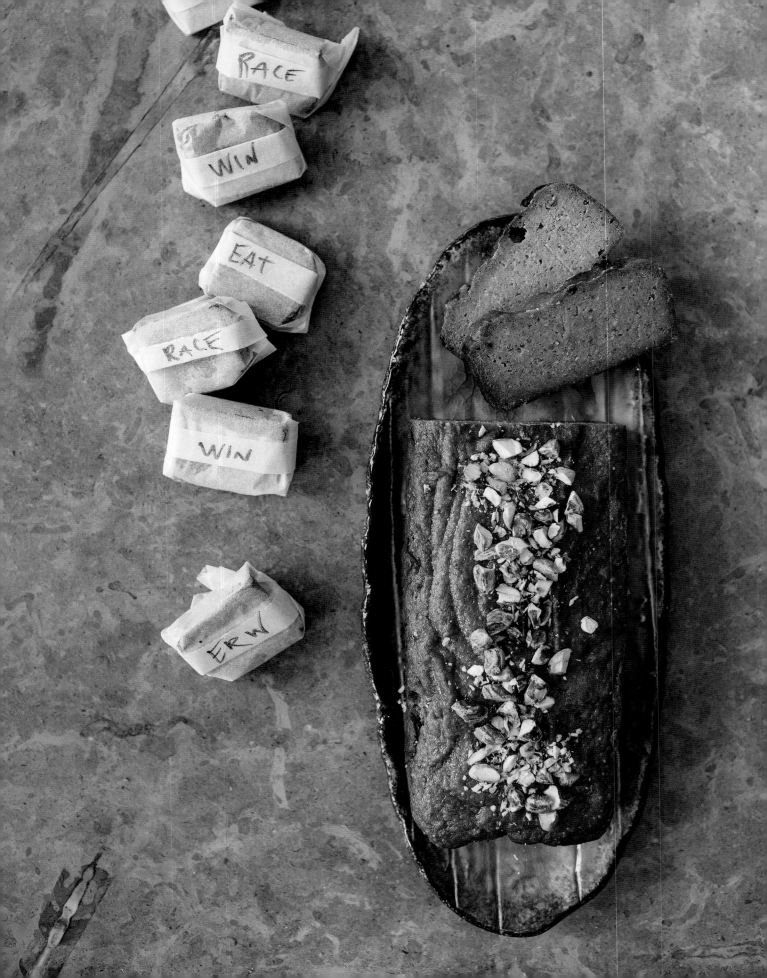

Flour-free Date and Fig Cake

Preheat the oven to 165°C/330°F. Grease a cake pan. In the bowl of a food processor fitted with the S-blade attachment, process the dried dates and figs, water, orange zest and juice, spices and salt until well puréed. Add the eggs, one at a time, and process until smooth. Add the coconut oil and process until smooth. Remove the blade from the processor bowl and fold in the almond flour.

—

Transfer the batter into the prepared pan and bake for 35-40 minutes, until a cake tester or toothpick inserted into the center comes out clean. Remove it from the oven and set it aside on a wire rack to cool completely. To glaze the cake, pour the melted chocolate over the top and sprinkle the toasted nuts before serving. Slice and refrigerate for up to 3 months.

—

TIP: This cake is great for racing! To make it suitable for on-the-go consumption, instead of glazing the cake with chocolate, fold chocolate chips into the batter.

Yield: 12 pieces

200 g soft, dried and pitted dates

200 g soft, dried figs

100 mL boiling water

Zest and juice of 1 orange

2 tbsp. spice blend (ground cinnamon, cardamom, ginger, nutmeg, and all spice)

½ tsp. salt

6 whole large eggs

5 tbsp. coconut oil or butter

200 g almond flour

100 g dark chocolate, melted

Toasted nuts, to serve

Celebration Brownies

Preheat the oven to 165°C/330°F. Grease a square cake pan. In a small mixing bowl, whisk the eggs until smooth and set aside.
In another mixing bowl, combine the almond flour, baking powder, and salt, then set aside. In a medium saucepan over low heat, combine the sugar, chocolate, butter and vanilla seeds.
Melt the mixture, gently stirring until completely combined.
Remove the saucepan from the heat. Gradually add in the whisked eggs; stirring until smooth. Fold the dry ingredients into the mixture until just blended.

———

Transfer the batter into the prepared pan and bake for 25 –30 minutes. When the core of the cake is still a little bit wobbly, remove the pan from the oven. The brownies will remain soft and chewy once they cool completely in the refrigerator.

———

TIP: This brownie has been served as a celebratory treat at many grand tours in the past. It has been tested and approved by many pro riders!

Yield: 12-16 pieces

5 whole large eggs

100 g almond flour

1 tsp. baking powder

1 tsp. salt

350 g brown sugar

340 g dark chocolate

170 g butter

1 vanilla bean

180 g chopped almonds or pistachios

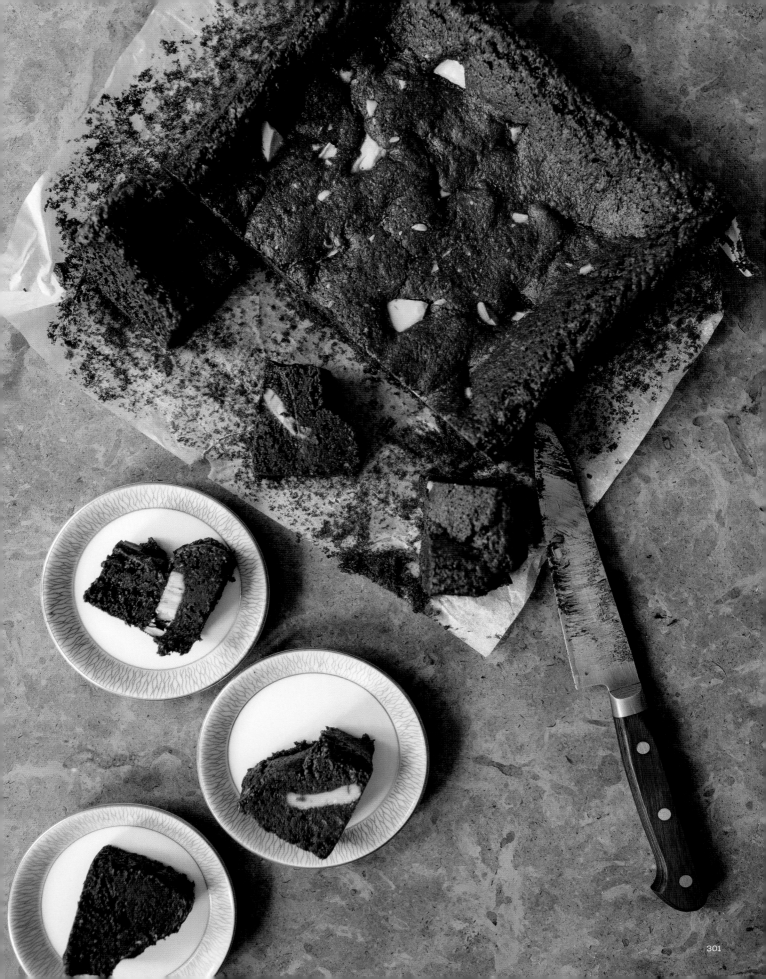

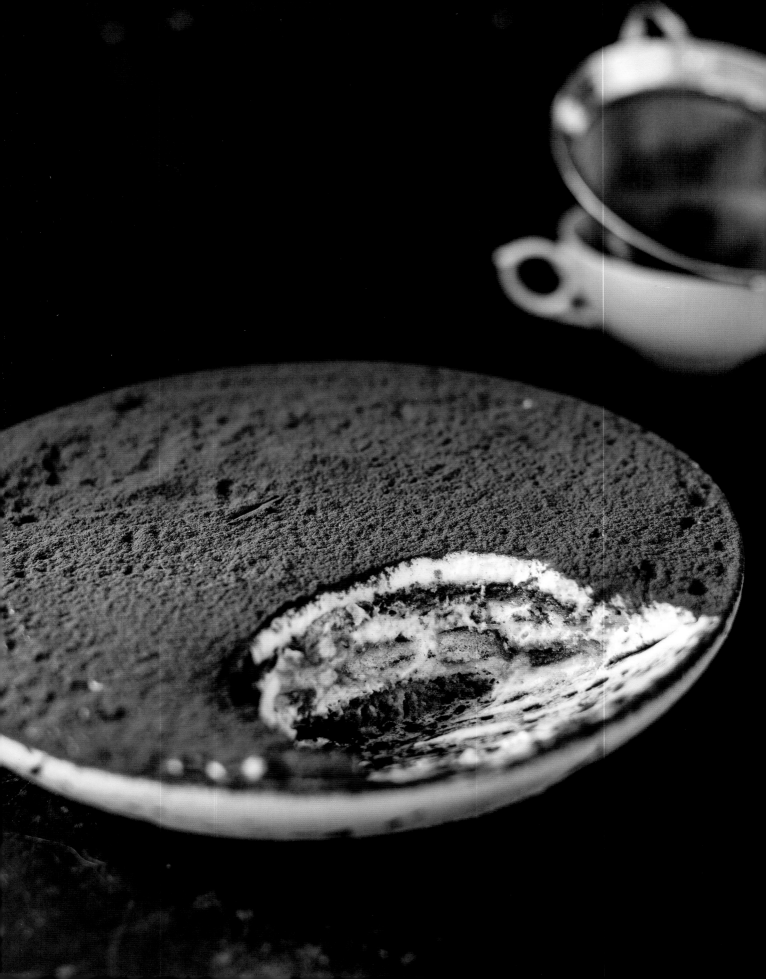

Winning Tiramisu

Preheat the oven to 180°C/355°F. Line a square metal cake pan with parchment paper, then grease and flour both pan and paper. Set aside a deep, narrow dish for tiramisu assembly.

To prepare the sponge cake: In a mixing bowl, beat the eggs and sugar together until foamy and white. Sift the flour into the bowl and gently fold it into the egg mixture. Transfer the batter into the prepared pan and spread it evenly. Bake it for 10–15 minutes until golden and set, then let it cool down completely on a wire rack. Slice the cake into 1.5 cm–thick strips that would fit the assembly dish.

To prepare the mascarpone filling: In a small mixing bowl, combine the mascarpone and 3 tbsp. of cream, then whisk them together carefully until smooth. In a second mixing bowl, beat the egg yolks and sugar together until foamy and white. In a measuring cup, soak the gelatin in the water for 30 seconds. Squeeze the excess water out and add the lukewarm espresso, then stir until combined. Whisk the remaining 250 mL of cream by hand until silky and smooth. To achieve the best result, the cream should be a little less whipped than optimal. Gently fold the mascarpone mixture into the egg yolk mixture until smooth. Fold in the gelatin mixture, then fold in the whipped cream.

To assemble the tiramisu: Stir the cold espresso and port wine together. Layer the base of the assembly dish with 1 strip of sponge cake. Drizzle some cold espresso mixture over the strip, then top it with a layer of mascarpone filling. Continue layering in this order until the dish is full. Cover with plastic wrap and refrigerate until it cools down completely. Dust with cocoa powder before slicing and serving.

TIP: To make it lighter, substitute mascarpone for thick 10% greek yogurt. Tiramisu is best enjoyed on day 2, so keep that in mind to prepare in time for celebrations and festivities!

Yield: 12-16 portions

Sponge Cake

4 whole large eggs

110 g granulated sugar

110 g all-purpose flour

Mascarpone Filling

250 g mascarpone cheese, at room temperature

3 tbsp. + 250 mL heavy whipping cream, divided

4 large egg yolks

3 tbsp. granulated sugar

3 g powdered gelatin

2 tsp. water

25 mL strong espresso, lukewarm

Tiramisu Assembly

200 mL strong espresso, cold

4 tbsp. port wine (for an extra festive feel!)

Unsweetened cocoa powder, to dust

Blondie "Chickpea Edition"

R G D V

Preheat the oven to 175°C/345°F. In a food processor, combine all the ingredients, except the chocolate, into a uniform paste. Mix half of the dark and white chocolates into the dough. Spread the dough out evenly onto a 20 cm x 20 cm cake pan. Press the rest of the chocolate into the dough and bake for 20-25 minutes until golden at the edges.

—

Let the cake cool down and cut it into 12 pieces. Serve as a delicious desert with berries and yogurt or divide into 12 and wrap individually as bars. Refrigerate for 3-5 days or freeze them for up to 3 months.

Yield: 12 portions

240g cooked chickpeas

65 g peanut butter

80 g maple/date syrup

1 big brown banana

50 g almond flour

½ pod vanilla

½ tsp. baking powder

75 g chopped dark chocolate

50 g chopped white chocolate

1 pinch salt

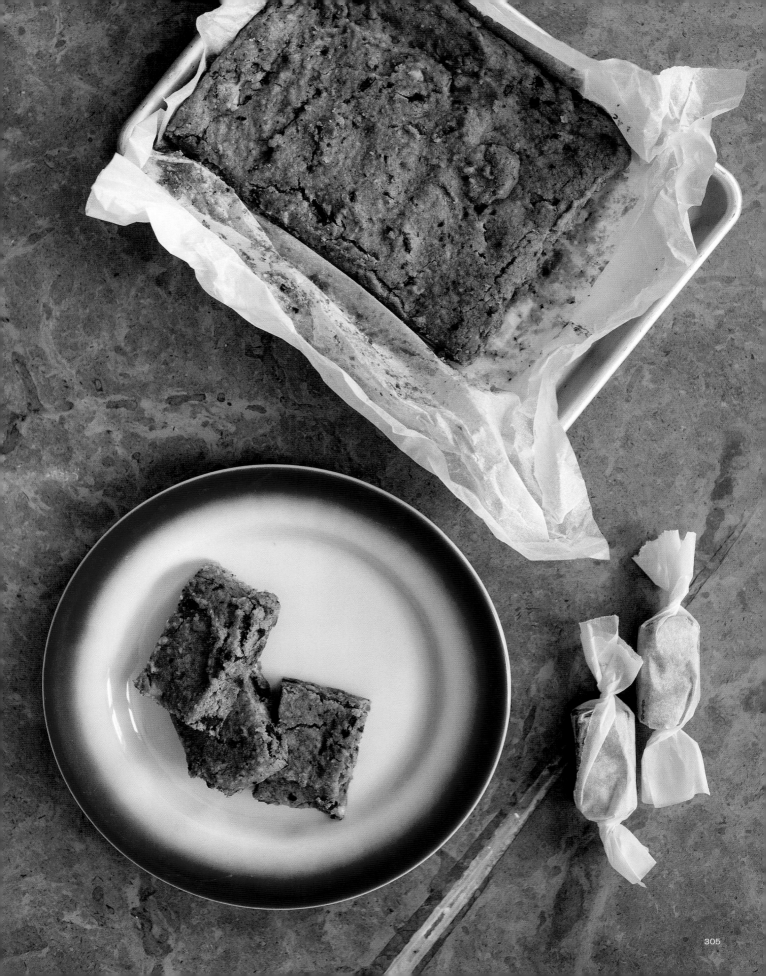

Race Bars, Balls and Bites

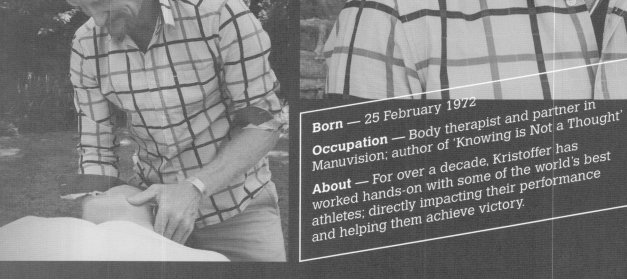

KRISTOFFER GLAVIND KJÆR

Born — 25 February 1972

Occupation — Body therapist and partner in Manuvision; author of 'Knowing is Not a Thought'

About — For over a decade, Kristoffer has worked hands-on with some of the world's best athletes; directly impacting their performance and helping them achieve victory.

"In intense endurance sports like cycling, proper fuel is not just important: it is paramount."

A Note from Kristoffer:

I've had the great fortune of working with Hannah Grant since 2010, when we were colleagues on a professional cycling team. Hannah's job was to provide the right fuel for the riders to endure the challenges of pro cycling, and mine was to prepare their bodies to be able to perform under the extremes of endurance.

My line of work is very much hands-on, with the goal being to optimize the body by making all its joints, tendons, and muscles work together as a unit. This work is very holistic in the sense that it focuses on many levels, right down to the well-being of specific organs and the importance of maintaining proper breathing.

Through this holistic approach, a whole new range of possibilities appears in order to unleash your specific potential. All of us are born with certain talents and skills, and in high performance sports, they're very easily measured. Your breathing capabilities (VO2 max), endurance, and strength (i.e. how many watts you can push out) are paramount. While there are some numbers we cannot change and what we're capable of is very much up to our DNA, we can still enhance the way our machine runs and recovers.

To improve our breathing, we can expand our thoracic region. We can also cleanse and nurture our organs so that they're better at digesting our fuel and turning it into energy. It may all sound very simple, but in reality, this means that the rider with the best recovery is the one who wins the long-stage races. The Giro, Tour de France and the Vuelta are 3 weeks of torture and agony, where just one off day could mean that you drop from 1st to 15th place!

The liver is vital for recovery and generating energy. In fact, its role is so complex and integrated in every process of the body that it's hard to overestimate its importance. Modern medicine has created artificial kidneys, lungs and even hearts, but to my knowledge, science has yet to come up with a substitute for the liver. When it's working well, it spends its time detoxing, rebuilding our system and making more energy, but when it has to use all of its resources to function, then it has less ability to help with recovery and give us power.

Toxins that digest slowly like alcohol, medicine, trans fats, and so on can start to build up if our intake is higher than what our body can cope with. Being an intelligent system, the body then stores them where they can do the least damage, that is, away from the vital organs and in the connective tissues, joints, and sometimes, even the muscles. This makes performance suffer in the long-run, in that you can have the strongest legs in the peleton, but if your machine is suffering, you will eventually get 'heavy legs', which is something every rider fears!

Hannah's cooking supports the liver and provides it with all that it needs to recover. More importantly, it avoids all the things that are hard on the liver. Eating a proper diet is detoxifying in itself, and by using anti-inflammatory ingredients, her food gives the immune system a real boost.

I got to experience this first-hand, because there was a big difference between the races when riders got the normal 'hotel buffet' food and the races where Hannah's food truck was around. During the long-stage races, it became especially clear that we had fewer infections and runny noses because the riders had better immune systems. For me as a 'body nerd', the biggest benefit was that their engines seemed smoother, and their muscles - more fit and agile.

Working with pro riders is like working with Ferraris in human form, where problems show themselves quickly. We can feel if the liver is blocked or if the bowels aren't performing properly. Due to the love Hannah poured into her cooking, the riders had decreased lactic acid and water retention after a mountain stage; and in the long-run, they needed less detoxification and experienced better recovery. Riding a race like Paris-Roubaix is hard enough as it is, and you don't want to push your luck by being constipated or choking from an overblown stomach.

Eating Hannah's proper balanced diet also decreased the amount of acid in the riders' bodies and increased the ability of red blood cells to obtain oxygen. The respiratory system is a complex process in which the amount of H+ ions plays an important role, where the more H+ ions (acid) there are in the body, the more oxygen we have to inhale. This means that if we eat a lot of acidic food, we need to balance the body with respiration, leaving less oxygen for the muscles to absorb.

In intense endurance sports like cycling, triathlons, and cross-country skiing, proper fuel is not just important: it is paramount. There may be many great chefs out there in performance sports, but Hannah's cuisine has something that performance cooking often lacks: a great sense of taste! Eating is one of the few pleasures allowed when competing at elite levels, and Hannah is at the forefront of bringing proper nurturing and tasty food to the world of pro cycling.

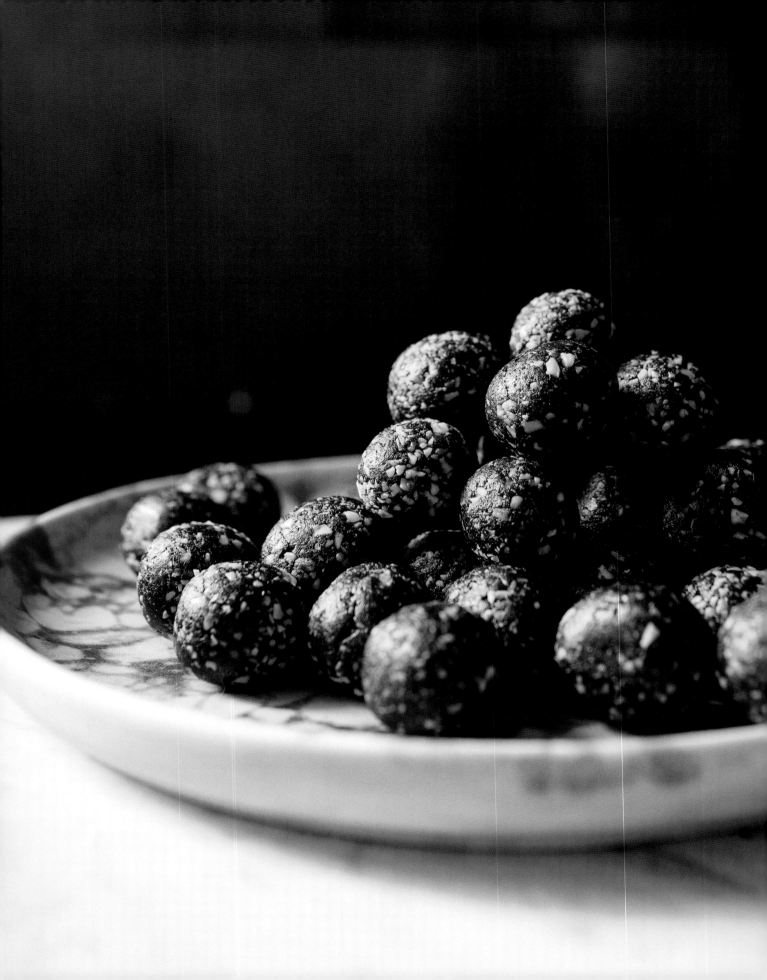

Caffeine Hit Balls

Combine everything in a food processor with the S-blade attachment. Roll into balls or shape as desired. Refrigerate in an airtight container for up to 2 weeks or freeze for up to 3 months.

—

TIP: Add a scoop of natural protein powder into the food processor for a boost! If you are using liquid coffee, increase the amount of nuts and cocoa powder slightly for better consistency.

Yield: 50-60 pieces

140 g raw almonds

125 g pecans

600 g medjool dates

80 mL very strongly brewed coffee or 2–3 tsp. instant espresso

50 g cocoa powder

1 tsp. pure vanilla extract

½ tsp. sea salt

Cookie Dough Chocolate Chip Bars

G D V

Combine everything except the chocolate chips in a food processor with the S-blade attachment. Add the chocolate chips and pulse 2-3 times. Press the dough into a plastic-wrapped container, let it cool down, and cut into bars or roll into balls. Refrigerate in an airtight container for up to 2 weeks or freeze for up to 3 months.

Yield: 40 pieces

160 g. rolled oats

2 tbsp. chia seed

280 g almonds

½ tsp. salt

½ tsp. cinnamon

25 g natural protein powder

600 g medjool dates, pitted

2 tbsp. coarse cane sugar

80 g dark chocolate, chopped

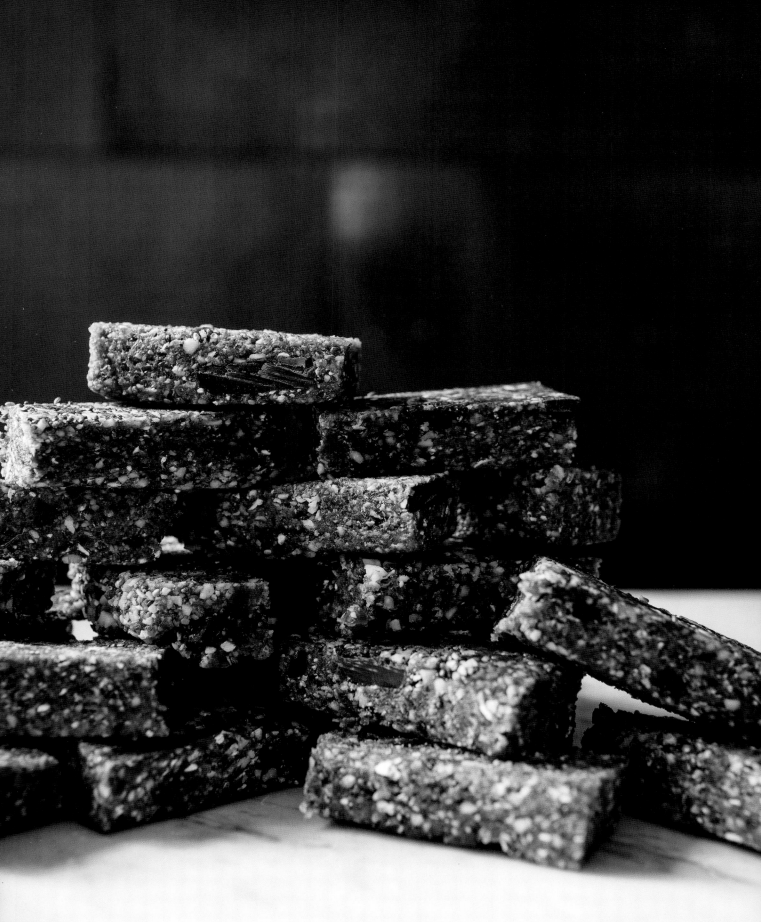

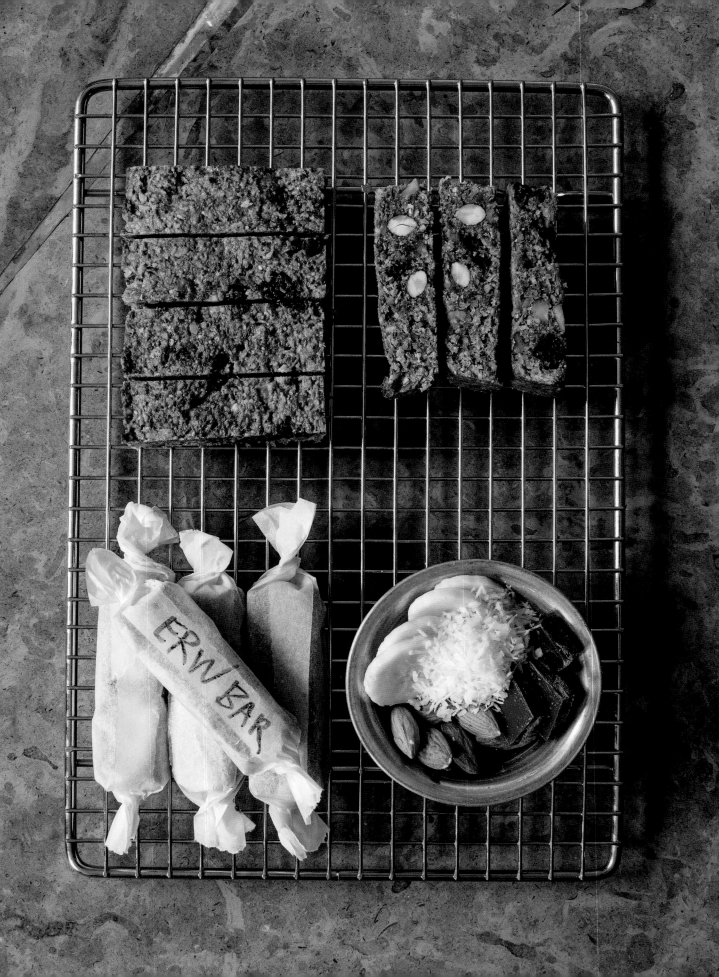

Baked Banana Bars

Preheat the oven to 175°C/350°F. Line a square baking tin with parchment paper. Blend or grind ⅓ of the oats into flour, then combine all the dry ingredients. Add the mashed bananas and other wet ingredients to the dry mixture, then combine well. Pat the mixture into the baking tin and bake for about 30 minutes until golden and firm. Let it cool down before slicing into bars. Refrigerate in an airtight container for up to 2 weeks.

—

TIP: Add a scoop of natural protein powder into the dry mixture for a boost!

Yield: 20 pieces

80 g rolled oats

65 g chopped walnuts

30 g shredded coconut

3 tbsp. chia seeds

45 g chocolate chips

¼ tsp. cinnamon, all spice or ginger powder

¼ tsp. fine sea salt

2 bananas, mashed

125 g peanut butter

85 g maple/date syrup

Coconut Rice Squares

G D V

Cook the sticky rice with the water in a rice cooker or in a pot covered with plastic wrap and a lid over low heat for about 60 minutes. In a separate pot, bring the coconut milk, sugar and salt to a boil, then simmer for 15 minutes. Add the cooked rice to the coconut milk and cook over low heat until most of the liquid has been absorbed.

—

Press the mixture into a container with parchment paper or plastic wrap. Let it cool down completely before slicing into squares. Refrigerate in an airtight container for up to 1 week.

—

TIP: For variations, add flavors, fruits, nuts, or seeds to your liking before pressing the mixture.

Yield: 20 pieces

450 g sticky rice

500 mL water

500 mL thick coconut milk

250 g brown sugar

1 pinch salt

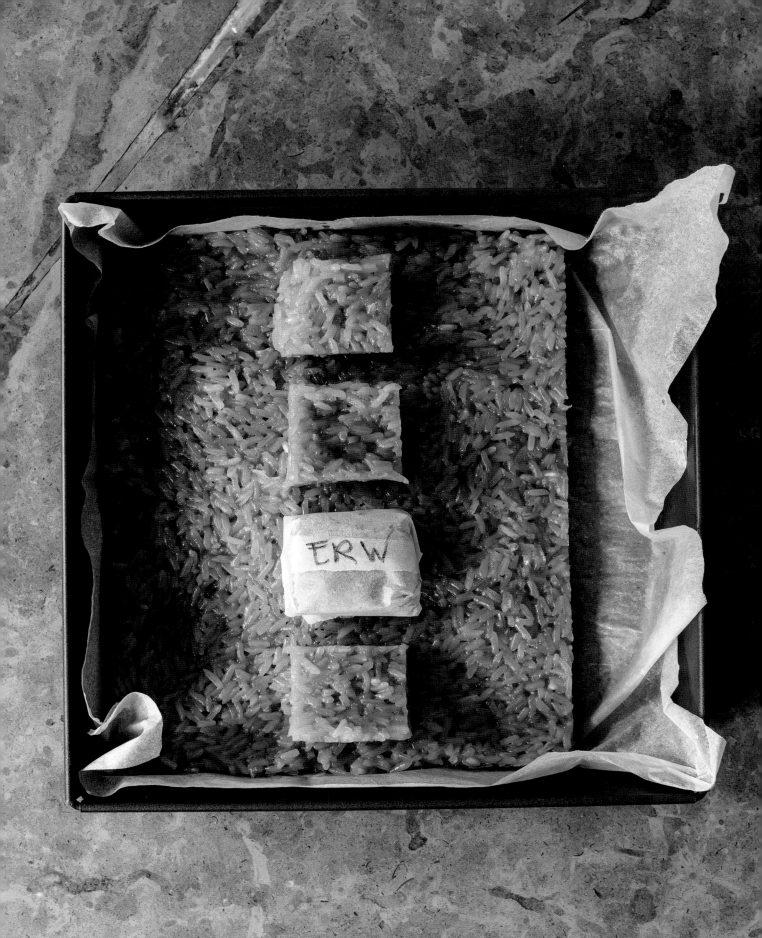

Sauces, Dressings and Broths

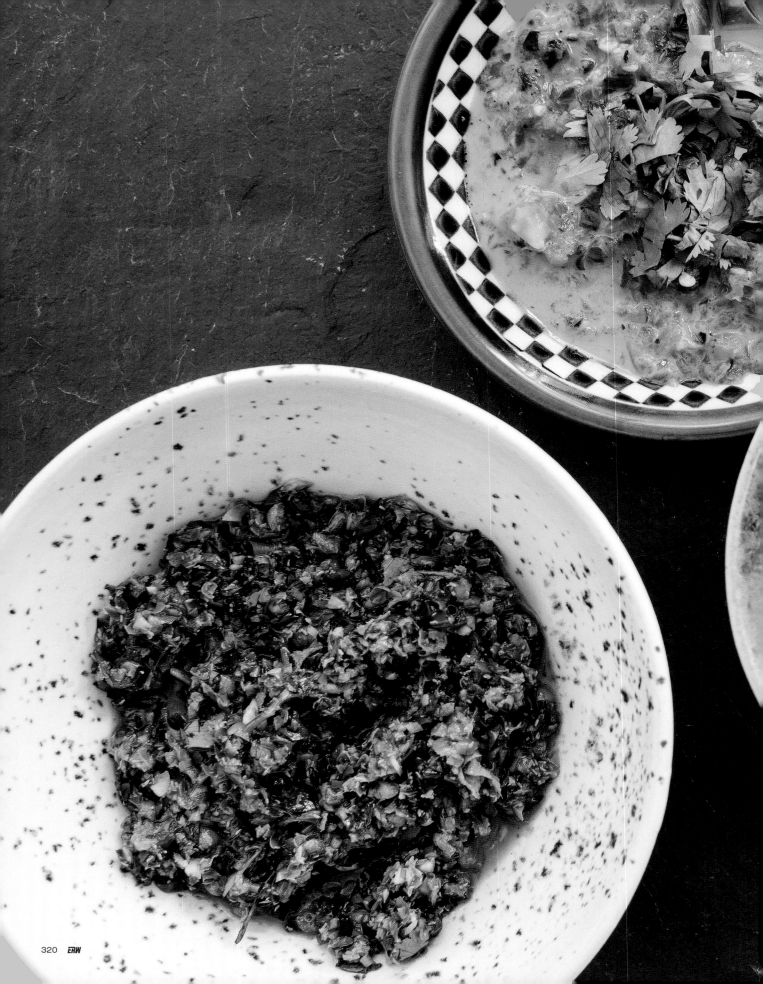

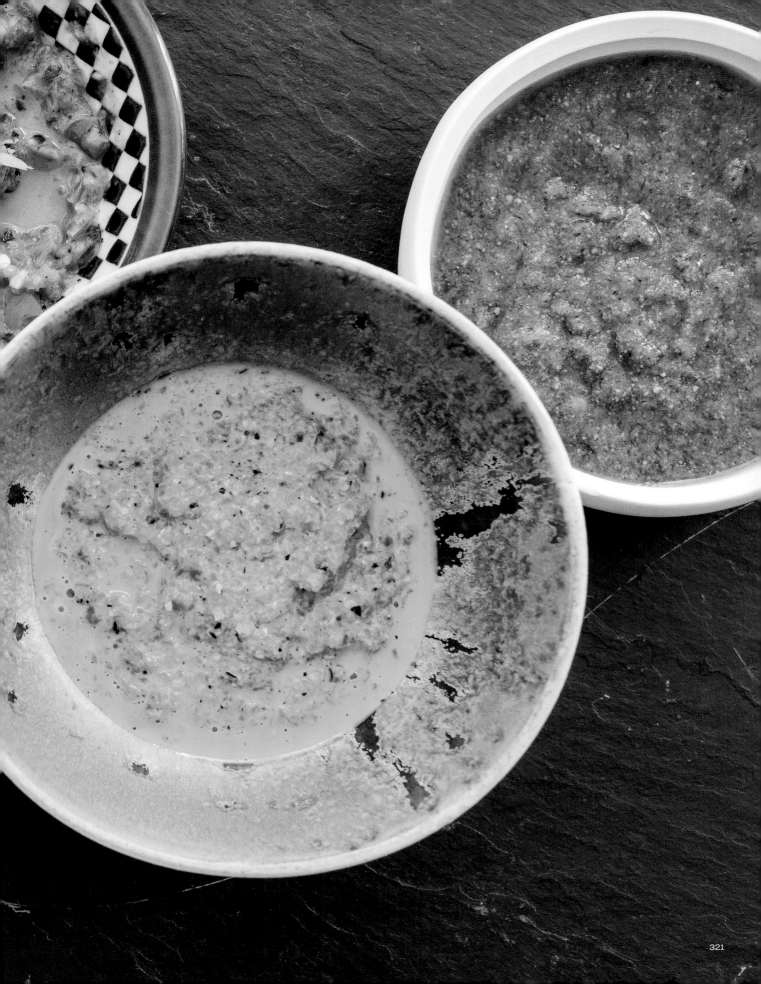

Basic Vinaigrette

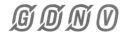

As long as the basic measurements are kept, you can make thousands of different dressings with this basic recipe!

Combine everything but the olive oil together. Whisk in the olive oil bit by bit until the dressing is thick and emulsified.

TIP: For variations, switch the apple cider vinegar with any desired type of vinegar. Add fresh herbs, berries or finely chopped nuts or seeds.

Yield: 30+ servings

200 mL apple cider vinegar

600 mL olive oil

1 tsp. salt

2 tbsp. Dijon mustard

1 tbsp. honey

Pepper, to taste

Green Herb Pesto

In the jug of a powerful blender, combine the herbs and garlic. While the blender is running, drizzle in the olive oil, then add the pine nuts and Parmesan. Season the pesto with the lemon zest and juice, as well as the salt and pepper to taste.

TIP: For variations, consider toasting the pine nuts or using seeds instead. You can also substitute the Parmesan with any hard cheese.

Yield: 20 servings

250 g mixed fresh green herbs (arugula, basil, flat-leaf parsley, chives, etc.)

1 clove garlic

200 mL olive oil + more if needed

100 g freshly grated Parmesan cheese

50 g pine nuts, almonds, hazelnuts or walnuts

Zest and juice of 2 lemons

Salt and pepper, to taste

Roasted Red Pepper Sauce

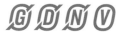

Heat up a pan with 1 tbsp. of olive oil. Roast the peppers over high heat until dark brown and tender. Add the garlic and sauté for 1 minute more. Add the water and bring to a boil, then remove the pan from the heat.

Transfer the sauce into the jug of a powerful blender and blend until smooth. While the blender is running, drizzle in the remaining oil and season with the salt, pepper, lemon zest and juice, as well as the chili pepper (if using) to taste.

TIP: For variations, serve with chopped fresh coriander, cilantro or parsley leaves.

Yield: 10+ servings

50 mL olive oil, divided

3 medium red peppers, seeded, cored, and sliced into thin strips

1 clove garlic, peeled and sliced

50 mL water

Salt and pepper, to taste

Zest and juice of 1 lemon

Fresh chili pepper, finely chopped (optional)

Olive, Capers, and Garlic Vinaigrette

Ⓖ Ⓓ Ⓝ Ⓥ

Combine all the ingredients except the olive oil and stir until well combined. Whisk in the oil and season with the salt and black pepper to taste.

Yield: 10+ servings

50 g green olives, pitted and chopped

50 g capers, in water

2 cloves garlic

Zest and juice of 2 lemons

1 bunch fresh flat-leaf parsley, rinsed, dried and roughly chopped

1 bunch fresh chives, rinsed, dried and roughly chopped

Salt and pepper, to taste

Anchovies, chopped (optional)

400 mL olive oil

Tomato and Oregano Salsa

Ⓖ Ⓓ Ⓝ Ⓥ

Season the tomatoes with the salt and black pepper. Combine all the ingredients, then season again to taste.

Yield: 8 servings

4 ripe tomatoes, shredded or grated

½ bunch fresh oregano, finely chopped

1 clove garlic, peeled and pressed

Salt and pepper, to taste

50 mL olive oil

Chimichurri Sauce

Ⓖ Ⓓ Ⓝ Ⓥ

Combine all the ingredients, then season with salt and pepper to taste. Stir until well combined. Cover it with plastic wrap and refrigerate for at least 3 hours (or overnight) to allow the flavors to meld.

Yield: 15+ servings

200 mL olive oil

100 mL red wine vinegar

½ bunch oregano, finely chopped

½ bunch fresh flat-leaf parsley, finely chopped

½ bunch fresh coriander or cilantro, finely chopped

1 medium shallot, finely minced

1 small chili pepper, finely minced

2 cloves garlic, finely minced

Salt and pepper, to taste

1-hour Chicken Broth in a Pressure Cooker

This is the fastest way to make broths. It is simple, and you can adjust the flavor to your liking by adding herbs, dried spices, and root vegetables. The flavor of any soup, sauce, or braising dish that requires water can easily be enhanced if you use broth instead.

For a basic broth: Bring bones and water to a boil in the pressure cooker. Skim the surface and close the lid. Bring the pressure cooker up to a high pressure, then turn it down and let it sit at a low pressure for 1 hour. Pull the cooker aside from the heat and let the pressure cooker cool down. When the pressure valve has gone down, open the lid. Strain the broth and skim away impurities. Use it as is or reduce it down to a more concentrated stock.

For a flavored broth: Follow the same procedures as the basic broth, but add a selection of flavor givers to the bones and water at the beginning. Flavor givers include carrots, celery, celeriac, onions, garlic, mushrooms, tomatoes, fennel, thyme, parsley, dill, rosemary, coriander seeds, peppercorns, star anise, fennel seeds, dill seeds, cinnamon, cloves, lemon zest, orange zest etc. Mix the flavor givers to your liking. Make sure to peel and clean them well. Use them raw or caramelize the surface to enhance flavor.

TIP: Refrigerate it in clean airtight containers or freeze for up to 3 months.

Yield: ~1.5 liters

Chicken scraps and bones from 1 chicken or more

Enough water to cover the scraps and bones without going above the security line in the pot

Basic Chicken Broth in a Pot

Use the same ingredients as the 1-hour broth. Flavor the broth to your liking with veggie scraps, and dried herbs and spices. Bring everything to a boil, skim away impurities, then turn it down to a simmer for 2 hours. Continue skimming the broth as it reduces and taste it as you go along. If you are making a very large portion, increase cooking time. Strain the broth at the end, bring it to a boil, and skim it again. Refrigerate it in clean airtight containers or freeze for up to 3 months.

Yield: 1-3 liters

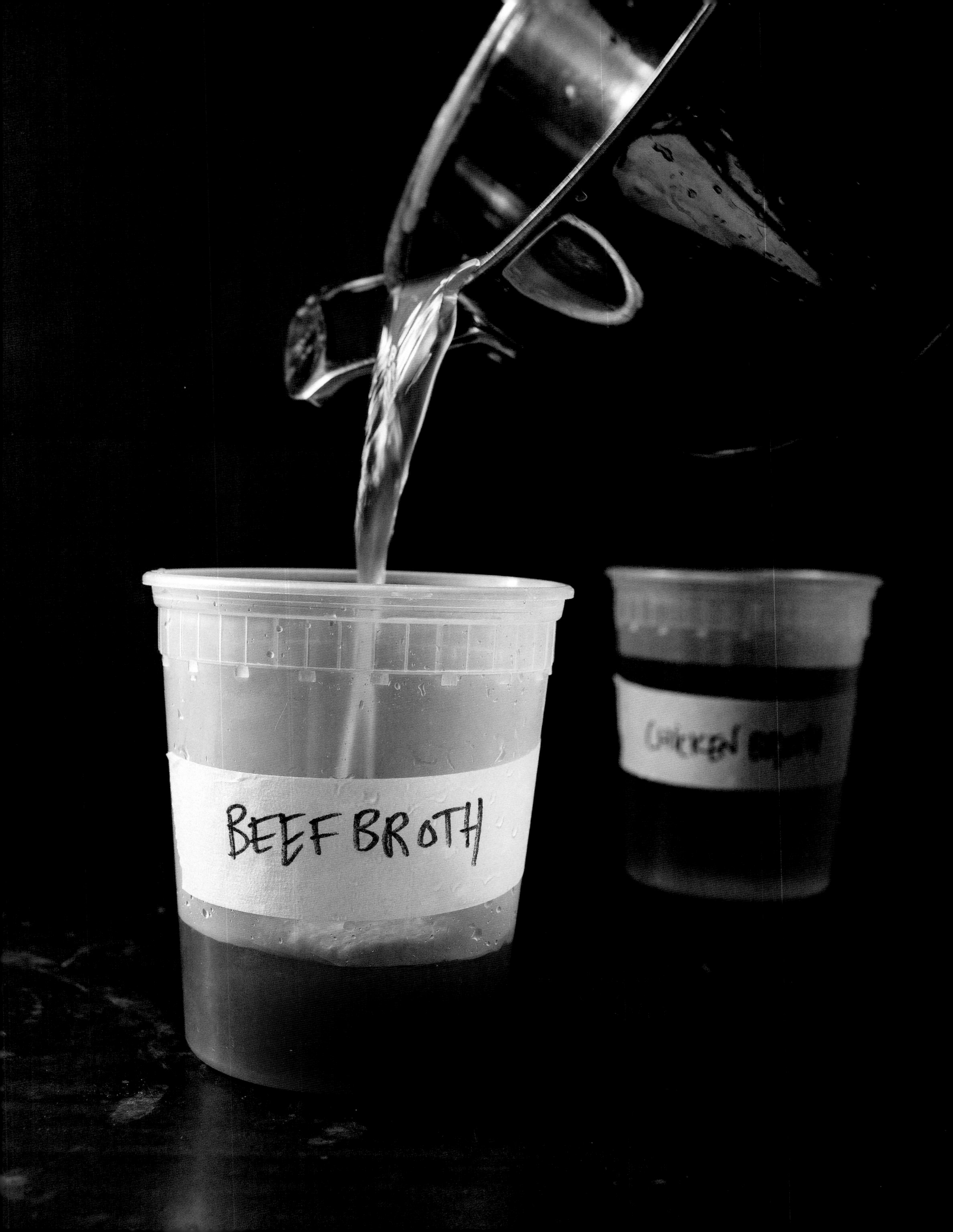
BEEF BROTH
CHICKEN

3-hour Beef Broth in a Pressure Cooker

Preheat the oven to 200°/395°F. Roast the beef bones until golden brown. Bring the bones and water to a boil in the pressure cooker. Skim the surface and close the lid. Bring the pressure cooker up to a high pressure, then turn it down and let it sit at a low pressure for 2 hours. Pull the cooker aside from the heat and let the pressure cooker cool down. When the pressure valve has gone down, open the lid. Strain the broth and skim away impurities. Simmer for 30 minutes and reduce it down to a more concentrated stock. Refrigerate it in airtight containers or freeze for up to 3 months.

TIP: Ask your butcher specifically for bones for broth. He can cut them into smaller pieces to fit in your pressure cooker.

Yield: ~1.5 liters

Beef bones

Enough water to cover the bones without going above the security line in the pot

Flavor givers (as explained in the 1-hour chicken broth recipe)

Basic Beef Broth in a Pot

Use the same ingredients as the 1-hour broth. Flavor it to your liking with veggie scraps, and dried herbs and spices. Bring everything to a boil, skim away impurities, then turn it down to simmer for 2 hours. Continue skimming the broth as it reduces, and taste it as you go along. If you are making a very large portion, increase cooking time. Strain the broth at the end, bring it to a boil, and skim it again. Refrigerate it in clean, airtight containers or freeze for up to 3 months.

Yield: 1-3 liters

A-Z Recipe INDEX

Ⓖ Gluten Free

Ⓝ Nut Free

Ⓡ Recovery

Ⓡ Race Food

A-Z Index ingredients

There is one person on the top of my list, without whom this book would not have been possible - my business partner and mentor, Mr. Ilya Katsnelson:

Dear Ilya, the amount of gratitude that I have for what you have done for me cannot be measured. I am forever grateful for how you mentor me, how you support me, and how you push me to always keep going and work through the tough times as well as the good times. You are the reason that I can share what I truly love doing with the world. Thank you, Ilya - from the bottom of my heart. I feel so lucky that you have chosen to believe in me, and work with me.

Next up is my trusty army of besties - Avalo, Christense, Sarah Backer, and Anna:

I love you all and thank you for being there for me - through the good times (with and without the wine and doggies), as well as the bad times when sh*t hit the fan. You ladies have a special place in my heart, and I count my lucky stars everyday for having you around me. Also, thank you for being my food guinea pigs... Christense, you have taken one for the team and probably eaten half of the meals in this book - AND approved of them!

Then, there is the one and only Mr. Christof Bove:

Dear Christof, you are by far the only person on the planet who has flipped my world upside down by taking me through countries, continents, altitudes, wild waters and sandstorms - both physically and mentally. Thank you for believing in me, and for bringing me to the next level. If only I knew what it would all lead to! Writing this in May '18, it is the calm before the storm, but let the adventures go on. There is never a dull time when I'm around you. ☺

Thank you to my amazing friends/colleagues/soldiers who have been working with me in business and life: Kristoffer-jazz omelet, Mentor mama Louisa Lorang, Sanne mor, Staven, Kristian Gajol pastil Baumann, Simis-Simon Krüger, Jonis Zeuthen Knoll, Denny-Benny Wang og Theis Maaaaaa.

Life is just more fun and awesome with you guys in it!

Keith, thank you for your advice, coaching and all the good times (and those to come)!

Lastly, but absolutely most importantly, to my mom Jette:

Dear Mom, thank you for being my motivation, and for teaching me that life is best lived when traveling. Thank you for giving me freedom within responsibility; for telling me to pursue my dreams and not settle down before I have done what I wanted to do. Thank you for always supporting me, for believing in me, for dealing with me, for listening to me, for hugging me, for feeding me, for giving birth to me. Tak mor, jeg elsker dig over alt på jorden.

Thank you!